Medical Advisory Board

Hope and Help
for Chronic Fatigue
Syndrome

The Official Guide of the CFS/CFIDS Network

Karyn Feiden

A Fireside Book
Published by Simon & Schuster
New York   London   Toronto   Sydney   Tokyo   Singapore

FIRESIDE
Simon & Schuster Building
Rockefeller Center
1230 Avenue of the Americas
New York, New York, 10020

1   3   5   7   9   10   8   6   4   2

Library of Congress Cataloging in Publication Data is available

ISBN 0-671-75944-2

This book is dedicated to the basic human right of accessible, affordable, and appropriate health care and to the hope that someday that right will be extended to all Americans.

Acknowledgments

Thanks goes first and foremost to all the physicians, scientists, and patients who took the time to speak with me about their experiences with chronic fatigue syndrome. A lengthy list of sources is included below.

Several physicians and patient experts read and commented on the manuscript. Dr. Paul Levine of the National Cancer Institute, a part of the National Institutes on Health in Bethesda, Maryland; Dr. Elizabeth Connick of Columbia Presbyterian Medical Center in New York City; and Dr. David Bell, who is in private practice in Lyndonville, New York helped assure the accuracy and comprehensiveness of the book. Gidget Faubion, former head of the Chronic Fatigue Immune Dysfunction Society, who was involved in this project from the earliest stages of development, Orvalene Prewitt, president of the National Chronic Fatigue Syndrome Association, and Marc Iverson, president of the Chronic Fatigue and Immune Dysfunction Syndrome Association in Charlotte, North Carolina also critiqued the manuscript and provided invaluable suggestions.

Two superb health care resource libraries deserve special mention. The Plane Tree Health Resource Center in San Francisco, California, and the Center for Medical Consumers in New York City have a storehouse of information on almost all health-related subjects and this book could not easily have been written without them. Both libraries are open to the public at regularly scheduled hours; their addresses are included in Appendix B.

My ever-alert agent, Barbara Lowenstein of Lowenstein Associates, first suggested a book on chronic fatigue syndrome, and my editor, Paul Aron, and P. J. Dempsey, now of Paragon Books, played crucial roles in making it a reality.

Deepest gratitude also goes to my family and to David, for his wisdom and his love.

Sources

The following physicians provided information for this book in both personal interviews and at scientific conferences:

Dr. Dharam Ablashi, herpes virologist, Laboratory of Cellular and Molecular Biology, National Cancer Institute, National Institutes of Health, Bethesda, Maryland.

Dr. David Bell, pediatrician, private practice. Associated with the University of Rochester Medical Center and Roswell Memorial Park Cancer Institute, Lyndonville, New York.

Dr. Nathaniel Brown, chief, pediatric infectious diseases, North Shore University Hospital. Associate professor, pediatrics and microbiology, Cornell University Medical College, Manhasset, New York.

Dr. Paul R. Cheney, senior staff physician, Department of General Internal Medicine, Nalle Clinic, Charlotte, North Carolina.

Dr. Richard E. DuBois, infectious disease specialist, internal medicine, Atlanta Medical Associates. Associate clinical professor, Medical College of Georgia, Atlanta, Georgia.

Dr. Jay Goldstein, family medicine, private practice, Anaheim Hills, California. Director, CFS Institute, Beverly Hills, California.

Dr. Robert A. Hallowitz, family medicine, private practice, Gaithersburg, Maryland.

Dr. Glen Hammer, infectious disease specialist, internal medicine, private practice, New York, New York.

Dr. Edwin J. Jacobson, internist and nephrologist, private practice. Associate clinical professor of medicine, University of California at Los Angeles School of Medicine, Los Angeles, California.

Dr. Carol Jessop, internist, Fairmount Medical Group, El Cerrito, California. Associate clinical professor, Department of Medicine, University of California, San Francisco, California.

Dr. James F. Jones, staff physician, Department of Pediatrics, National Jewish Center for Immunology and Respiratory Medicine, associate professor of medicine, University of Colorado School of Medicine, Denver, Colorado.

Dr. Anthony L. Komaroff, chief, Division of General Medicine, Brigham and Women's Hospital. Associate professor of medicine, Harvard Medical School, Boston, Massachusetts.

Dr. Paul Levine, senior investigator, Environmental Epidemiology Branch, National Cancer Institute, National Institutes of Health, Bethesda, Maryland.

Dr. Stephen Marlowe, infectious disease specialist, internal medicine, Atlanta Medical Associates, Atlanta, Georgia.

Dr. Phil Pellett, virologist, Centers for Disease Control, Atlanta, Georgia.

Dr. Neil Singer, internist, private practice. Clinical instructor, Mount Zion Hospital, San Francisco, California.

Dr. John Stewart, virologist, Centers for Disease Control, Atlanta, Georgia.

Dr. Stephen Straus, chief of medical virology, Laboratory of Clinical Investigation, National Institute for Allergy and Infectious Diseases, National Institutes of Health, Bethesda, Maryland.

Dr. Leonard S. Zegans, professor of psychiatry and chairman of the education department of psychiatry, University of California at San Francisco, San Francisco, California.

[ ]

A number of other health professionals offered distinct and valuable perspectives on chronic fatigue syndrome and the challenge of coping with prolonged illness:

Ricki Boden, social worker, Operation Concern, San Francisco, California.

Sharon Kaplan, social worker, Mt. Sinai Medical Center, New York, New York.

Nancy Durkin, board member, National Council on Independent Living, Bethel, Connecticut.

Valerie Kistler, supervisor, Policy Management Section, Disability Program, Branch Office of the Regional Commission of the Social Security Administration, Boston, Massachusetts.

[ ]

Without the commitment and energies of support group leaders and political activists around the country, the struggle to bring chronic fatigue syndrome to the forefront of public attention would not have been possible. Even as they struggled with illness themselves, they organized patient support groups, medical conferences, and congressional letter-writing campaigns, called media attention to the problem, sponsored fund-raising drives, and sought to persuade a skeptical medical community of the legitimacy of their illness.

The following CFS activists spoke with me during the preparation of this book:

Catherine Beason, New York, New York

Janet Bohanon, Kansas City, Kansas

Condy Eckerle, New York, New York

Evelyn Eisgram, New York, New York

Barbara Humphreys, Atlanta, Georgia

Marc Iverson, Charlotte, North Carolina

Gidget Faubion-Jones, Portland, Oregon

Bob Landau, Elizabeth, New Jersey

Ken Lipmann, New York, New York

Jan Montgomery, San Francisco, California

Orvalene Prewitt, Kansas City, Missouri

Nick Richmond, New York, New York

Barry Sleight, Washington, D. C.

Mimi Tipton, Wilmington, Delaware

Theodore Van Zelst, Chicago, Illinois

Dozens of other patients all over the country shared their personal stories with me. At their request, the names have been withheld to protect their privacy but this book has been greatly enriched by their candor.

About the Sponsor:
The CFS/CFIDS Network

Without the commitment of a loyal cadre of patient act.vists, it is uncertain when chronic fatigue syndrome (also known as chronic fatigue and immune dysfunction syndrome, or CFIDS) would have gained the attention of the national press and the scientific community. Beginning in 1981, when the CFIDS Society first opened its doors ir. Portland, Oregon, patients have played a leading role in bringing credibility to the illness and providing relief to the countless thousands who suffer from it.

Today, three national organizations devote themselves to educating the public about chronic fatigue syndrome. Joining the Portland organization are the CFIDS Association in Charlotte, North Carolina, which publishes the *CFIDS Chronicle,* and the National CFS Association in Kansas City, Missouri. All three patient advocate groups field media inquiries, encourage research, and provide direct assistance to patients and their families.

The support of all three groups was crucial to this book:

Chronic Fatigue Immune Dysfunction Syndrome Society
P.O. Box 230108
Portland, Oregon 97223
Yvonne Alderman, Office Manager
(503) 684-5261

Chronic Fatigue and Immune Dysfunction Syndrome Association
P.O. Box 220398
Charlotte, North Carolina 28222
(800) 44-CFIDS and (900) 988-CFID
Marc Iverson, President

National Chronic Fatigue Syndrome Association
3521 Broadway, Suite 222
Kansas City, Missouri 64111
(816) 931-4777
Janet Bohanon, Orvalene Prewitt, Co-Directors

Contents

Introduction

David S. Bell, M.D., FAAP

Last fall, en route to Newport, Rhode Island, for a national scientific conference on chronic fatigue syndrome, my car began to sputter and falter, refusing to maintain a steady speed. The problem worsened steadily and eventually I pulled into a small-town garage, where I slept fitfully until a mechanic came on duty the following morning.

The mechanic tinkered cheerfully with my car, checking the fuel line, electrical system, and various other parts but could not find anything wrong. We drove the vehicle around the block together and this time it ran perfectly. "Wish I could tell you what the problem is but I just can't see it," he said. "I'd keep a close eye on it and stop again as soon as it starts acting up."

I was struck by this incident because it contrasted so markedly with the prevailing attitude of the medical community toward chronic fatigue syndrome. Physicians, it seems, have forgotten how to say "I don't know." Unlike my mechanic friend, they often become suspicious about symptoms they don't understand and defensive toward illnesses they cannot cure. Instead of viewing a new problem as a challenge—and meeting it with original research and creative thinking—some doctors explain away enigmatic sicknesses with inappropriate labels like "depression" and "psychosomatic disorder."

Few patients have paid a higher price for this failing than those stricken with chronic fatigue syndrome. CFS, formerly called chronic Epstein-Barr virus syndrome and a host of other names, is a common and frequently devastating illness. As described so vividly in this excellent book, thousands of patients present their physicians with a multitude of symptoms, pay hefty fees for sometimes painful diagnostic procedures, and end up with a bewildering array of faulty and even absurd explanations. Medical insurance coverage for many procedures is spotty and patients who are unable to work may lose what health insurance they have. Social Security disability payments are hard to obtain and emotional support is often absent altogether.

Chronic fatigue syndrome patients deserve better. Much of the progress that has been made in our understanding of this illness can be traced directly to their educational and organizational efforts. It is ironic that millions of patients have learned to analyze the significance of medically arcane findings about natural killer cells and interleukin-2, while many physicians are still debating whether the illness exists at all. We owe our patients more than just healthy skepticism; we also owe them compassion and a commitment to work harder to understand what ails them.

My own experiences with chronic fatigue syndrome have convinced me that it is an organic medical illness. In Lyndonville, New York, an upstate farming community, I was a firsthand witness to an epidemic of CFS, which struck in October 1985. Some 150 people in this sparsely populated region have since been diagnosed with the mononucleosis-like illness. Children have been particularly hard-hit: Sixty young people under the age of eighteen, most of whom had previously been completely healthy, now suffer the symptoms of CFS. The limitations of medical understanding and the sometimes overwhelming needs within our community have propelled me into further involvement with this illness. Today I am absorbed in scientific efforts to understand the etiology, epidemiology, and pathology of chronic fatigue syndrome, particularly as it affects children, and I work closely with researchers and patient support groups from around the country.

Dr. Paul Cheney, one of the first physicians to recognize this disorder, recently said to me, "CFS is initiating twenty-first century medicine." I have no doubt that he is right. Over the past two hundred years, most medical diagnoses have been made on the basis of individual organ failure. CFS defies this approach, for despite extensive patient complaints, pathology reports show no tissue damage. To understand this complex, multisystem illness, we must instead couple state-of-the-art technology with our increasingly sophisticated understanding of the immune system. For the researcher willing to tackle this exasperating illness, the payoff is the opportunity to unravel once unsolvable medical mysteries.

The next best thing to a cure for CFS is patient and physician education. An informed patient can assume increased responsibility for obtaining appropriate treatment and banish doubt about the validity of the illness. An informed physician can provide empathetic and appropriate healthcare and make referrals to the range of other support services patients need. By explaining complex medical concepts coherently and presenting the full range of debate on the illness objectively, *Hope and Help for Chronic Fatigue Syndrome* helps provide that badly needed education.

Dr. David S. Bell is medical director of the World Life Institute, which studies health, nuclear radiation, and toxic waste issues. He is also associated with the University of Rochester Medical Center and Roswell Memorial Park Cancer Institute and is involved with chronic fatigue syndrome research and advocacy efforts around the country.

PART I

What Is Chronic Fatigue Syndrome?

■

An Illness Emerges:
Overview of Chronic Fatigue
Syndrome

I think what we are faced with is the problem of defining a new
disease. There is need for multidisciplinary approaches. We are talking
about a disease, the investigation of which requires epidemiologists,
immunologists, virologists, psychologists. Why the psychologist? To
prove you're not all crazy.

> –Dr. Seymour Grufferman, Pittsburgh Cancer
> Institute, Pittsburgh, Pennsylvania

This is probably the most interesting disease I have ever encoun-
tered because it is so complicated, it deals with so many different
systems of the body. It is exciting to be working on a new disease,
the way it must have been at the turn of the century, when the
microbe hunters were just beginning to discover that bacteria actually made people sick.

> –Dr. Jay Goldstein, CFS Institute, Beverly Hills, California

Chronic fatigue syndrome (CFS) burst into public consciousness in the
1980s. Unexpected as a tornado and almost as devastating, CFS rips
apart the lives of its victims, often incapacitating them in the prime of
life while shattering personal relationships and destroying careers. The
illness is causing alarm within the scientific community and hardship
and heartbreak among the afflicted.

What is this demonic illness that is wreaking such havoc? It has
been easier for physicians to say what chronic fatigue syndrome is not
than to explain what it actually is. It is not mononucleosis, although
profound fatigue is its most uniform marker. It is not Alzheimer's

disease, although patients often report the periodic confusion and memory loss associated with that grim disease. It is most assuredly not AIDS, although there is evidence of immune system abnormalities. Nor is it anemia, multiple sclerosis, lupus, rheumatoid arthritis, or Hodgkin's disease, but it has sometimes been confused with each one of these.

A skillful imitator, chronic fatigue syndrome is a debilitating illness in its own right. It often strikes suddenly, then lingers stubbornly for years. According to a background piece issued by the National Institutes of Health, the federal agency known as the Harvard of biomedical research:

> The hallmark of the illness is fatigue—a fatigue that comes on suddenly and is relentless and relapsing, causing debilitating tiredness or easy fatigability in someone who has no apparent reason for feeling this way. Unlike the mind fog of a serious hangover, to which CFS has been compared, the profound weakness of CFS does not go away with a few good nights of sleep but instead slyly steals a person's vigor over months and years.

Along with an exhaustion that leaves many people bedridden, frequent CFS symptoms include headache, muscular and joint pain, sore throat, balance disorders, sensitivity to light, an inability to concentrate, and quirky, inexplicable body aches. Symptoms wax and wane in severity and linger for months, sometimes years, while ambitious professional and personal plans grind to a halt. The roller-coaster pattern of sickness makes planning impossible and often taxes the patience of the most compassionate friends and relatives. Effective treatment remains elusive and there is no cure.

But the prognosis is not altogether grim. Many patients eventually do recover, although some must operate at a reduced level for years afterward. It is rare that the illness progresses to something more serious and there have been no documented fatalities.

The story of Sharon M.'s struggle to overcome her illness is typical. Sharon, age thirty-four, was an economics professor at a Chicago university before she was felled:

> I've been battling with this thing for two years. My career and my social life are still on hold. Sometimes I wonder if I'll ever be entirely well again.
>
> I still remember the day I awoke with a sore throat and an aching body. I've never been the same since. During my worst periods, the exhaustion was simply indescribable. It was an effort to talk on the

telephone and doing household chores was impossible. Dragging myself to the bathroom sapped me of energy for an afternoon. Making the rounds of doctors was a nightmare beyond imagination. At first, no one could identify my ailment. I saw internists, allergists, neurologists, and gastroenterologists. The severity of my symptoms didn't match the findings of conventional laboratory tests and I sensed the physicians' disbelief. The kinder ones talked candidly about psychosomatic illness and told me to lower my level of stress. Others said flatly they could do nothing for me except recommend a good shrink.

I was discouraged, depressed, and beginning to doubt my own sanity. But after I had been sick for a year I read an article in the local newspaper that described a woman whose illness sounded very much like mine. I called her and then saw the doctor she recommended. After examining me thoroughly, he confirmed the diagnosis of chronic fatigue syndrome.

I remember how elated I was that day. Although the doctor told me there was no known cure, all I cared about at the time was that he acknowledged the legitimacy of my sickness. I still have a long way to go before I'm well but at least I understand what's wrong with me now.

Although patients with CFS are understandably frustrated with the slow progress the medical community has made toward a full understanding of their illness, recent developments actually provide reason for optimism. A few short years ago, little was known about the diagnosis, cause, or treatment of chronic fatigue syndrome, researchers were doing almost no work in the field, and no public monies had been allocated for further study. The predictable result was that patients were frequently misdiagnosed, encouraged to undergo costly and inappropriate laboratory tests, accused of malingering, or simply shunted aside by a medical community that did not understand them.

Thanks in good measure to the dedicated work of patients themselves, CFS has clearly emerged from that bleak period of neglect. Tremendous strides are now being made. Researchers in prestigious laboratories around the country are engaged in path-breaking studies and the scientific knowledge accumulated in recent years about the immune system, viruses, and the physiological effects of stress has begun to enrich our understanding of CFS. Although a cure is only a distant hope, physicians are experimenting with treatment regimens to relieve symptoms and boost overall function. Perhaps most important, the hard-won credibility now accorded CFS means that patients need not feel alone or abandoned any longer.

For the History Books

In the annals of recent CFS history, three key events are remembered for their role in galvanizing the attention of the American medical community and the popular press. In 1984, rumors of a mystifying illness began to circulate in a Nevada resort community. The following year, medical journals carried reports of patients exhibiting symptoms similar to those observed in Nevada and suggested a viral cause for them. And in 1988, four years after the first epidemic was reported, a federal agency defined chronic fatigue syndrome for a worried public.

Incline Village, Nevada, 1984:
An Epidemic Erupts

Incline Village, Nevada, has a well-earned reputation as a playground for the well-to-do. Lapped by the waters of Lake Tahoe, its resorts attract skiers in the winter and recreational boaters in the summer. Indifferent to the seasons, the gamblers flock to the nearby casinos year-round. The mountain air is invigorating here and the pollution-free skies are backdrop to a universe of stars.

It seems an unlikely setting for an epidemic. And internists Paul Cheney and Daniel Peterson initially thought nothing terribly amiss when patients trickled in complaining of exhaustion and a hodgepodge of other vague symptoms. But month after month their patient load kept growing and by the end of the fateful year of 1984, the trickle had become a flood. Patients did not respond well to conventional treatment and no one seemed to be getting much better. Curiosity slowly turned to alarm. The problem seemed to be spiraling out of control.

Laboratory tests intended to pinpoint the cause of the severe symptoms came back relentlessly normal but Drs. Cheney and Peterson never doubted the word of their patients. Both men had worked in the community for many years and had known many of their patients when they were in the pink of health. These are not hypochrondriacs, they agreed. But a painstaking search of the medical literature provided no easy explanation of cause or suggestions for treatment and both physicians felt stumped.

Is the Epstein-Barr Virus the Culprit?

The first break in the Incline Village enigma came in January 1985, although research had actually been completed prior to the Nevada outbreak. Two path-breaking articles were published that month in the *Annals of Internal Medicine,* a widely respected medical journal that reports on scientific research and chronicles major medical breakthroughs. The articles described chronically ill patients struggling with overpowering fatigue and speculated that active infection with the Epstein-Barr virus, a herpes virus known to cause mononucleosis, was the cause.

"An important feature of this patient group was a degree of disability seemingly out of proportion to the objective extent of the illness. By all regards, including formal evaluations, many of these patients appeared to be neurotic. However, our detailed studies have uncovered a series of subtle yet objective, organic abnormalities in these patients," wrote Dr. Stephen E. Straus of the National Institutes of Health and his coauthors in one of the two seminal papers. "Several features of the disease and the laboratory abnormalities suggest that Epstein-Barr virus may underlie the disorder . . . The disorder we are considering to be chronic Epstein-Barr virus infection is not rare and warrants further investigation. For now, it is of immeasurable benefit to patients with this disorder to document an organic basis for their complaints."

Bingo, thought scores of physicians scouring the medical journals for an explanation of what they were seeing in private practice. Aha, sighed resolute patients sloughing through highly technical articles in search of an explanation their physicians could not provide, perhaps *that's* what's ailing me.

The articles reached a wide audience and phones around the country started to ring. Physicians called patients and said, "I've got a theory as to what might be ailing you. Can you come in to be tested for the Epstein-Barr virus?" The diligent Cheney-Peterson medical team got word of the research and tested their Nevada patients for evidence of an active E-B infection—and detected extraordinarily high antibody levels in one-third of them. When the media picked up the story, newspaper headlines and television reports alerted isolated and frightened patients all across America of the new findings.

Ironically, the thesis that Epstein-Barr virus is directly implicated in chronic fatigue syndrome has since been sharply questioned by researchers, including some of the original authors of the *Annals* articles. Experts from the Centers for Disease Control (CDC), the Atlanta-based federal agency charged with safeguarding the public health, investigated the Incline Village epidemic and concluded that Epstein-Barr might not be the sole culprit after all. Nonetheless, the Nevada outbreak and the subsequently published research marked the first time scientists and physicians began to pay serious attention to the disorder—and the moment that patients around the country realized they no longer had to suffer in silence.

An Official Definition at Last

Under pressure from Congress and patient support groups around the country, the Centers for Disease Control released a long-awaited clinical definition of chronic fatigue syndrome in March 1988. In doing so, lead author Gary P. Holmes, an epidemiologist in the CDC's Division of Viral Diseases, and fifteen other top researchers and clinicians took an enormous stride toward eliminating any lingering skepticism about the legitimacy of the illness. Their article, which appeared in the *Annals of Internal Medicine,* is designed to ensure that any research data generated on CFS is consistent and comparable.

In brief, the CDC definition calls for the exclusion of a long list of conditions—from AIDS to schizophrenia—whose symptoms are sometimes confused with chronic fatigue syndrome. In addition, patients must demonstrate persistent and debilitating fatigue and as many as eight other specified signs and symptoms, including fever, muscle or joint pain, headaches, neuropsychological problems, swollen lymph nodes, and sore throat, over a period of at least six months. A detailed summary of the CDC definition is provided in Appendix A of this book.

The definition was officially drafted for research purposes, although primary-care physicians are also relying on it as an aid to reach diagnosis. The guidelines are deliberately specific so that scientists can learn as much as possible about a relatively small patient population. "Persons who may have less severe forms of the syndrome or who have less characteristic clinical features may be excluded by the new definition," write the authors, acknowledging that it is certain to be revised as more information becomes available.

With a formal definition to guide them, researchers now know they will be comparing similar patient populations—eggs to eggs, rather than eggs to apples. Meaningful epidemiologic studies can get underway as a result and our knowledge about the number and types of people with CFS is sure to be vastly expanded over the next few years. By following a given patient population over time, we will also be able to learn much more about the waxing and waning of symptoms, how many patients fully recover from illness, and whether other medical problems are likely to present themselves in the future.

What's in a Name?

Ever since the first outbreaks of chronic fatigue syndrome were widely reported in the mid-1980s, the illness has been shrouded by doubts and often mistaken for depression or neurosis. The uncertainty about its true nature is reflected in the lingering controversy over the name, which Boston researcher Dr. Anthony Komaroff—paraphrasing Winston Churchill's famous remark about democracy as a form of government—called "the worst possible name except for all the rest."

Chronic Epstein-Barr virus syndrome, or CEBV, was the name of choice in the mid-1980s, after the virus was fingered in the Incline Village epidemic and in the first *Annals of Internal Medicine* articles. Once the Epstein-Barr virus was ruled out as the certain cause, the Centers for Disease Control hit upon chronic fatigue syndrome and that name has been adopted by the U.S. Public Health Service, the Congress, and some of the patient support groups.

But not everyone is satisfied. Most patients feel it trivializes the illness. The national patient organization in Charlotte, North Carolina, was the first to refer to the illness as chronic fatigue and immune dysfunction syndrome (CFIDS) in the belief that it more accurately reflects the true nature and severity of the illness. Throughout Europe, myalgic encephalomyelitis, or ME, is preferred. More generally, the illness has been called postviral fatigue syndrome, because many physicians believe it is the result of a lingering viral infection. Other labels include chronic mononucleosis; neuromyasthenia, meaning nerve and muscle disease; and sometimes chronic, epidemic, sporadic, or postinfectious neuromyasthenia.

Regardless of its current-day moniker, most knowledgeable scientists believe that an illness akin to chronic fatigue syndrome has been with us for centuries. The medical literature describes epidemic outbreaks for at least fifty years. Many came to be known according to their geographical setting—for example, Icelandic disease, after an epidemic was reported in Iceland in 1948, and Royal Free disease, named for a 1955 outbreak at the London Royal Free Hospital.

The best retrospective study of these and other outbreaks comes to us from England. *Postviral Fatigue Syndrome: The Saga of Royal Free Disease* is written by Dr. A. Melvin Ramsay, one of the first investigators to scrutinize the epidemic at the Royal Free Hospital, where 292 medical and administrative staff members fell ill. Along with a detailed account of the London outbreak, Dr. Ramsay looks back through medical history to uncover some fifty-two reports of similar epidemics in the past fifty years. Washington, D.C., Florida, Greece, Scotland, South Africa, and several English towns, including Coventry, Middlesex, and Newcastle upon Tyne, were among the afflicted locales. Following are some of the incidents that made the headlines of their day:

• In 1934, at Los Angeles County General Hospital, almost 200 medical personnel were crushed by overpowering fatigue, muscle weakness, memory lapses, and sleep disturbances. More than six months after the epidemic peaked, 55 percent of the victims were still unable to return to work.

• Just a few months after it had been wracked by a polio epidemic in May 1949, a CFS-like illness plundered the community of Adelaide, Australia. Over an eighteen-month period, some 700 individuals were hospitalized for treatment.

• An epidemic swept through a convent in New York State in 1961. Along with the familiar symptoms of exhaustion, impaired thinking, and body pain, many of the ailing nuns reported a burning sensation when they swallowed and numb or tingling hands, arms, and legs.

• In the 1980s, several provincial towns in Scotland reported an epidemic pattern of illness characterized in part by acute vertigo, anxiety, muscle twitching, and ringing of the ears, as well as extreme fatigue. Women—ranging in age from eight to fifty-three—outnumbered men by more than two to one.

In the United States, the Incline Village story helped make the obscure Epstein-Barr virus a household word, but it is only the decade's best-known cluster outbreak. Similar stories have been heard elsewhere. Pediatrician David Bell has extensively documented an epidemic among the rural residents of Lyndonville, New York. Cluster incidents have also been reported by members of an orchestra in North Carolina, students and teachers in a midwestern public school system, workers in a building in Ohio, and elsewhere.

While epidemics capture the most dramatic headlines, growing numbers of sporadic reports are equally alarming. Support groups operate in every state in the union and hundreds of articles on the syndrome have appeared in local newspapers from Maine to Alaska, clear indications that few communities are unaffected by the problem. In Rhode Island, public officials were so concerned about the impact of CFS on the state's economy that legislators financed a symposium for nationally recognized medical experts at which Governor Edward D. DiPrete and Senator Claiborne Pell both spoke movingly of the looming danger.

Despite the convincing claims of Dr. Melvin Ramsay and other researchers, we cannot be certain that the illness now wreaking havoc on the lives of so many of America's best and brightest is identical to past outbreaks. Dr. Paul Cheney has a particularly interesting perspective on this matter. "The concept of a postviral fatigue syndrome is probably as old as man and viruses," says the internist, noting, however, that the syndrome has historically been self-limiting (meaning that lingering signs of a viral infection ultimately disappear of their own accord). Only rarely have individuals been stricken by prolonged viral fatigue. And when epidemic outbreaks have been seen, they have traditionally been confined to a narrow geographic area.

This pattern of postviral fatigue is very different than what we are seeing today, according to Cheney, who observes: "What we have been seeing in the last fifteen years is common, prolonged, and appears to be generalized across national boundaries. And I don't think we have seen this before."

How Big Is the Problem?

Speculation that chronic fatigue syndrome is more widespread and longer-lasting than at any time in the past raises a basic and still unanswered question: How many people have it? Hard numbers probably won't be available for several years but it is likely that in the United States alone the ranks of the afflicted run to the millions. No respecter of national boundaries, cases of CFS have also been reported in England, Australia, New Zealand, Israel, and elsewhere.

There is plenty of evidence that the illness represents a major public health problem. Any time chronic fatigue syndrome receives publicity, whether on national television or in a community newspaper, there is a tidal wave of patient response. "I thought I was going crazy until I read about others like me," and "I never revealed how poorly I felt because I looked perfectly healthy and felt certain no one would believe me" are frequently heard comments. The National Institute of Allergy and Infectious Diseases, a branch of the National Institutes of Health, says that one-third of all inquiries received by its Office of Communications relate to chronic fatigue syndrome; only AIDS attracts a comparable volume. Local support group leaders say they are inundated with cries for help and voluminous requests for information from desperate patients and their families.

Doctors who have earned a reputation for compassionate and knowledgeable dealings with CFS patients also confirm fears that an epidemic is upon us—many say they are besieged by referrals and sometimes forced to close their doors to new patients. "Every day my office gets ten phone calls for me to see somebody," says Dr. Carol Jessop, an internist in the San Francisco Bay area who turns patients away when she cannot give them the intensive care and follow-up attention they require.

In 1988, the Centers for Disease Control launched a study to produce firm statistics. Soon afterwards, Walter J. Gunn, the principal investigator, had established a surveillance network in Atlanta, Georgia; Reno, Nevada; Grand Rapids, Michigan; and Wichita, Kansas—four cities whose populations are fairly representative of the nation as a whole in terms of age, racial distribution, and socioeconomic status. By 1991, preliminary results were already suggesting that the incidence of illness was much higher than expected.

Who Are the Victims?

The favored target of chronic fatigue syndrome is often previously healthy men and women with many interests and responsibilities. Although physicians have diagnosed children, teenagers, and people in their fifties, sixties, and seventies with CFS, the illness appears most likely to strike adults from their mid-twenties to their late forties. Women are afflicted anywhere from twice to three times as often as men, although there are indications that cases among men are rising. For reasons that remain unclear, the vast majority of the patients are white.

Curiously, a disproportionate number of healthcare workers, teachers, and people associated with the airline industry report the symptoms of chronic fatigue syndrome. The significance of this observation remains unclear but it does suggest avenues for further research—for example, researchers may want to look more closely at the environmental agents found at concentrated levels in airplanes, at chemicals frequently used in hospitals, and at the possibility that an infectious agent carried by children can cause more serious illness in adults.

Yuppie Flu: Fact or Fiction?

The age of many CFS patients, coupled with the fact that they are often affluent white professionals, prompted media wags to dub CFS the "yuppie flu" and "affluenza."

Admittedly clever turns of phrase, the names quickly took hold in the popular press, but to CFS patients the misnomers are symbolic of the cavalier attitude with which their illness is too often addressed. Condy Eckerle, a young New Yorker who has become a local watchdog of press coverage on the subject, remembers how he felt when he heard a radio program in which the pejorative phrase "yuppie flu" was used:

> At the time I was barely able to walk further than one or two blocks without reaching a state of total collapse and my body was so completely wracked with pain that I felt as if I just would not be able to bear another day of it. You can see why I felt insulted by his ingratiating little laugh, his lighthearted remark, and that utterly ridiculous epithet, the yuppie disease.

Dr. Carol Jessop theorizes that the myth of yuppie flu is linked to the battle to convince the medical community that the illness is legitimate. To persuade skeptical doctors that CFS is more than an illness of neurotic women, she has sometimes gone out of her way to portray patients as successful superachievers. "You say 'this woman is really together, she's got a great job, and she's earning lots of money—this isn't your garden-variety, depressed, hysterical woman.' You have to make that sort of preface so they understand they have to take this patient seriously."

While good health is universally valued, of course, some argue that high achievers are the most acutely aware of their illness simply because they need such high levels of energy. In the general population, the consequences of limitation may be less dramatic. Young professionals—accustomed to a lifetime of good health and physical fitness, to functioning at 100 percent of capacity and beyond and to realizing ambitious goals along the way—are not willing to go gently into the darkness of chronic illness. Nor do they readily accept a physician's skepticism and uncertainty. Hence the odyssey from doctor to doctor until diagnosis. "We're not willing to be written off as hypochondriacs," says Gidget Faubion, former head of the Oregon-based Chronic Fatigue and Immune Dysfunction Syndrome Society. "There are doctors trying to convince our patients that it is all in their heads and we just won't buy it."

The Gender Gap

It is thought that at least twice as many women as men suffer from chronic fatigue syndrome. One possible reason is that women are generally more prone than men to autoimmune disorders, such as lupus, multiple sclerosis, and rheumatoid arthritis, in which the immune system attacks the body's own tissue; some physicians suspect CFS is also linked to autoimmunity. The hormonal differences between the sexes could also prove to be a factor, either helping to prod a latent virus into attack or exacerbating the symptoms of illness. Or a sociocultural explanation could be involved: Women traditionally seek medical care more readily than men, especially for such amorphous complaints as fatigue.

Whatever the reason, some people believe that sexism has had much to do with the initial reluctance of the medical establishment to take chronic fatigue syndrome seriously. "Throughout history, there has been a pattern of refusal to recognize diseases that primarily affect women," says Jan Montgomery, the moving spirit behind the San Francisco CFIDS Foundation, which is seeking local public health funds to study and combat the illness. "We can believe that a bunch of Legionnaires get sick from air-conditioning but as soon as we talk about women and women's diseases we always want to start introducing the idea of stress."

The Racial Discrepancy

Although viruses seldom discriminate by race or socioeconomic class, most identified CFS sufferers are white. Dr. Richard E. DuBois, a physician who sees both a substantial number of chronic fatigue syndrome patients and a great many blacks in his downtown Atlanta, Georgia, practice, reports that there is practically no overlap between the two groups. "I can count on one hand the number of blacks I've seen with chronic fatigue," he says.

There are several possible reasons why. In minority communities, particularly poor ones, access to healthcare has always been marginal and physicians may simply be less likely to see this patient population. Given the ordeal that many patients endure before they are diagnosed, the ability to maneuver through a sometimes hostile bureaucracy may require skills more commonly found in a well-educated population.

Or genuine racial differences in the incidence of CFS may exist. One explanation centers on the likelihood that many black people are exposed to certain viruses when they are young. In urban areas, in impoverished communities, and within large families, children often come into contact with a wide range of viruses and thus develop the protective mechanisms they need to stave off acute infections as adults. Infectious mononucleosis, caused by the Epstein-Barr virus, is one example of this phenomenon. Because most blacks have been exposed to EBV as children, they rarely contract the so-called kissing disease that often afflicts white adolescents. We also know that certain viruses are much more virulent in older people: For example, an adult exposed for the first time to varicella zoster, which causes chicken pox, is much more likely to become seriously ill than a child. Thus it stands to reason that if a virus—or a combination of viruses—is ultimately implicated as a causative factor in CFS, blacks are less likely than whites to fall ill because they have already developed resistance to many viruses.

The Credibility Debate

While great strides have been made in the battle to give legitimacy to chronic fatigue syndrome, the disorder continues to engender a significant degree of skepticism, and sometimes ridicule. "Epidemic hysteria is a well-known problem," says one highly placed epidemiologist on the federal payroll. "We simply cannot address the problem of chronic fatigue syndrome in a scientifically rational way. The vagueness of this syndrome makes me feel as though I am chasing a ghost."

This kind of attitude persists despite the definition of the syndrome that has been released by the Centers for Disease Control. Doubt lingers even though the U.S. Congress has funded the first comprehensive epidemiologic study on chronic fatigue syndrome. Physicians continue to raise their collective eyebrows while potentially path-breaking experiments get underway at the National Institutes of Health and in hospital and university laboratories around the nation.

And perhaps most incredibly of all, suspicion takes no holiday even as patients with nothing to gain and everything to lose continue to seek medical treatment for this baffling illness. Writing in *The CFIDS Chronicle,* the newsletter of the CFIDS Society in Charlotte, North Carolina, president Marc Iverson wrote: "Too often because our illness does not 'fit the rules' we have been victims of an arrogant medical doctrine that holds 'if I can't diagnosis or understand your illness (and my technology can't detect it) it must not exist—or you must be psychoneurotic.' "

The impact of the lingering skepticism has had a devastating effect on many patients. Said one forty-year-old New Jersey woman, "I was told there was nothing physically wrong with me, that the symptoms were all in my head. I was accused of being a malingerer and a neurotic. How many times can one hear such accusations before starting to believe they must be true?" A man who journeyed to specialized clinics around the country in a three-year search for a diagnosis recalls, "It wasn't just that they didn't know what was wrong, it was that they didn't believe what I was describing to them. They dismissed my illness just because they didn't have the scientific data to understand it."

Why have so many patients been forced to endure such ordeals? There are a number of explanations. First, fatigue is one of the most common complaints that family-care physicians hear. Other accompanying symptoms, notably sleep disorders and panic attacks, resemble classic psychological depression and some busy physicians have leapt quickly to the conclusion that depression is what ails the patient. Dr. James Jones, an immunologist with the National Jewish Center for Immunology and Respiratory Medicine in Denver and a leading CFS researcher, told a local newspaper, "We're taught in medical school that if you can't put a name on it, it must be psychosomatic."

The fact that very few abnormalities can be uncovered by simple laboratory tests also adds to the skepticism. "Doctors need something they can detect and measure in order to diagnose a disease and they haven't known how to do this with chronic fatigue syndrome," says Dr. Jay Goldstein, a Los Angeles-based family physician with a particularly strong interest in CFS patients. A patient's appearance is rarely helpful, either; there is often no visible evidence of ill health.

Another factor contributing to the uncertainty surrounding CFS is the irrefutable fact that change comes slowly to the American medical establishment. Most physicians are understandably leery about anything they perceive as a "fad" disease until a great deal of well-documented and replicable research—judged valid by a highly critical jury of scientific peers—has been published in a select few medical journals. Such caution is certainly not all bad. 'You want physicians to be skeptical, not gullible," warned one doctor. The unfortunate result, however, is that today's CFS patients remain defenseless on the front lines of a mysterious illness while debate rages around them.

Within the next few years, this situation is likely to ease considerably. The CDC definition will enable researchers to sharpen their picture of chronic fatigue syndrome and conduct scientifically rigorous studies of proposed treatments. AIDS-related research is certain to yield a greater understanding of the astonishingly complex immune system and the workings of viruses. The expanding field of psychoneuroimmunology, which focuses on how the nervous and immune systems interact, will help us understand the organic impact of stress. Together these developments will stretch the frontiers of medical science and eventually shed some light on the enigma of chronic fatigue syndrome. In time, they will also enable physicians to understand what causes CFS, who is susceptible to its debilitating power, and what can be done to cure it.

Patient Power: Overcoming Skepticism and Building Support

Patients—the very same people whose energies have been sapped and whose professional and personal lives have been devastated—have been the most vocal advocates of their own cause. Without their determination and commitment, it is certain that far less progress would have been made in the struggle to combat chronic fatigue syndrome.

The groundswell of local and national activity follows the footsteps of the early days of the AIDS epidemic, when the gay community first organized to provide patient services and bring public attention to that cruel plague. Then, as now, government failed to respond to a crisis with due haste and a community of the afflicted arose to fill the ensuing gap. Then, as now, community activists learned that political bureaucracies are slow to respond to new problems and that effective organizing is necessary to prod them into action. And then, as now, public health departments and elected representatives eventually heard the cries for help from their constituents and began to allocate the funds necessary to combat a health threat of uncertain proportions.

The earliest organizing efforts took place abroad. Patient organizations such as ANZME (Australia-New Zealand Myalgic Encephalomyelitis Society) and the Myalgic Encephalomyelitis Association in England pioneered support group and advocacy work and served as important models for American activists. In the United States, Nomi Antleman of Tucson, Arizona, became one of the unsung heroines of the CFS movement. Her insistent efforts eventually awoke the media to the severity of the problem and nationally syndicated radio broadcaster Dr. Dean Edell ran one of the earliest programs on the issue. Shows on "20/20," "Nightline," "Oprah Winfrey," and elsewhere soon followed.

Meanwhile, awareness of the critical need for a national association began to build and activists in Portland, Oregon, stepped in to fill the void. More recently, major organizations in Charlotte, North Carolina, and Kansas City, Kansas, joined in the fray and hundreds of community-based groups have also emerged.

The Founding of the CFIDS Society

In Portland, Oregon, history was made in Martha Wolfe's living room in 1985. A group of patients—linked only by a set of peculiar symptoms that no doctor could explain—met to try to make sense out of the illness that was devastating their lives.

The story actually began some months before, when an article appeared in Portland's daily newspaper, *The Oregonian*. Author Martha Wolfe described the debilitating symptoms that forced her to quit teaching in an elementary school. The article struck a respondent chord in scores of local residents and Wolfe fielded so many inquiries that a meeting for all interested parties was organized. Participants recall the 1985 meeting as characterized principally by overwhelming relief: "I thought I was alone," was the common refrain.

From that first meeting emerged recognition of a widespread problem and the consensus that concerted, national action was needed to combat it. Within months, the groundwork for a formal nonprofit organization had been laid, and by September 1985, the Chronic Fatigue and Immune Dysfunction Syndrome Society, then known as the Chronic Epstein-Barr Virus Association, had opened its doors. From those humble beginnings, an international organization of patients, medical personnel, and concerned friends and family has evolved and continues to provide patient services, publish newsletters and fact sheets, and fight for research funds and credibility.

The Struggle Continues

Patient advocacy work has come a long way since that first meeting. The work has simply grown too large for one organization to handle and today numerous others are making important contributions as legislative and funding advocates, public relations experts, and sources of information and referral. Many of these organizations field inquiries from the press, maintain close contact with top researchers around the country, and counsel the sometimes frantic patients and concerned family members at the end of a long and desperate search to understand an illness their doctors cannot explain.

In Washington, D.C., patient advocates have worked to inform senators and congressmen about the growing public health menace of CFS and bolster funding. Both the ongoing Centers for Disease Control surveillance study and activities at the National Institutes of Health also reflect patient pressures. The NIH is currently conducting a long-term study of CFS patients at its Bethesda, Maryland campus, and has funded five additional research projects at universities. In March 1991, the NIH also sponsored a conference for CFS researchers around the country.

In Charlotte, North Carolina, the CFIDS Association issues a major monthly newsletter on the syndrome. Packed with articles discussing current medical thinking about cause, diagnosis, and treatment; describing patient group activities around the country; and analyzing holistic health remedies, the *CFIDS Chronicle* has become a key reference source for patients, physicians, and the interested public.

In Kansas City, Kansas, the National Chronic Fatigue Syndrome Association works to educate patients and their families, as well as health professionals and the public, about the nature and impact of CFS and to generate public and private research funds. An important information and referral source, the association provides guidance to new support group leaders, educational flyers for physicians, and a quarterly newsletter.

In Denver, Colorado, the Chronic Fatigue Syndrome Research Foundation has launched an ambitious project to raise funds for medical research. Along with major grants from corporations and institutions, the foundation works to raise money from patients themselves. In one fund-raising appeal, foundation representatives wrote, "No matter how large or small, every contribution to CFS research sends a loud, clear message to our lawmakers that CFS should be a priority issue . . . By contributing money to the future of your own health, you not only hasten the discovery of a cure but you vote to make CFS a national health priority."

In San Francisco, California, the Chronic Fatigue Immune Dysfunction Foundation has been notably successful in pressuring the city's public health department to make CFS a local priority. Now it plans to share its success by training patient leaders elsewhere in the nation in the art of political organizing, coalition building, and applying pressure to local decision makers.

Meanwhile, hundreds of support groups have sprung up in local communities around the nation. "Patients need each other," says Janet Bohanon, co-director of the Kansas City organization. "We are all living through this thing and we understand from the depths of our soul what it is like."

[   ]

While the panoply of symptoms differ from patient to patient, and the name is not everyone's first choice, there is no doubt that CFS is dramatically altering the lives of millions of Americans. And the danger seems to be drawing nearer: "Whatever it is, it seems to be growing in frequency," said Dr. Anthony L. Komaroff, chief of the Division of General Medicine at Brigham and Women's Hospital in Boston in an interview with the New York Times. "Literally every time I say to a friend that I'm studying this illness, and then describe it, they say 'Oh my God. My niece has it, or my next-door neighbor, or my boss.' "

In the following section, we'll meet some of the patients who have endured the ravages of chronic fatigue syndrome. Then we'll look at just what the scientific community knows about chronic fatigue syndrome thus far—and what possibly can be done about the debilitating illness.

Profiles: The Patients

Mimi Tipton

Mimi Tipton, age forty-one, can pinpoint almost the precise moment that she became ill. An account executive with a Wilmington, Delaware, telecommunications firm, she recalls: "On January 24, 1986, I was at work on an important proposal and all of a sudden I couldn't write anymore." Shortly afterward, her temperature soared to 105°F and the mental confusion that has been one of the hallmarks of her illness set in. By September, she had dropped 30 pounds, spent $10,000 on diagnostic tests, and taken a leave of absence from her job.

> The difference between me now and before the illness is like night and day. Now I accomplish less in one week than I did in one day. Last winter I accomplished less in one month. I used to read all the daily newspapers, *The Wall Street Journal* and the trade journals. After I got sick, I was lucky if I could read Ann Landers. There have been times when I don't have the strength to wash my hair or brush my teeth. And sometimes I'll have the strength to brush my teeth but I don't know how.

Despite her ravaged career and diminished acuity, Tipton has no time for self-pity. She has coordinated as many as six support groups at once in Philadelphia, Delaware, and southern New Jersey, and in a single year fielded 2,000 calls from patients, families, and physicians, most of them as she lay resting in the queen-size bed that doubles as her office.

> I went through a period of anger. I felt like a parasite because I had always been a productive member of society and now I was nothing. Then I started revising my priorities and setting realistic goals. I stopped competing with my old self.
>
> If you have the flu for a week or two, you have the luxury of feeling sorry for yourself, but with a chronic illness you've got to gain control of your reactions. I realize now that I can't do the things I could do before but I can do different things. It brings meaning to my illness to be able to help other people.
>
> One of the things I emphasize is the need to be patient. And hope is essential. When you lose hope, you lose a lot.

Bob Landau

Bob Landau knows his battle with chronic fatigue syndrome has irrevocably altered his life but the thirty-three-year-old blonde has effectively translated the lessons learned from his own pain into compassion for others. Warm, confident, and highly knowledgeable about his own illness, Landau has earned a reputation for leadership within both the New Jersey and New York support groups.

Until he became ill four years ago, the Ivy League school graduate was a transportation traffic rate analyst and a singer with the New York Choral Society, away from home six days and seven nights a week. "I was always running," recalls Landau. The onset of his illness came slowly, clouding his mind until he was unable to think straight. "I struggled on at work for a while but I would sometimes have to stop what I was doing and put my head down on my desk." He passed the first years of his illness in a fog, and at its worst, barely remembers the passage of time. Landau knows that he was bedridden for long spells, though, and gained 100 pounds as a result of the inactivity.

Private disability insurance, Social Security, Medicare benefits, and crucial help from friends and family enabled him to survive financially. Short-term therapy proved a vital tool for dealing with stress. But the biggest changes are coming now that he is well along the road to recovery. And Landau admits that he is frightened:

> For so long I've felt as though I was treading water in molasses and now I've got to get on with my life. It is scary to think of returning to the real world. And a new career is traumatic for anyone.
>
> But I'm happier now than before I got sick. Illness forces you to make a lot of changes and change is always difficult, but it can be interesting. One thing I've realized is that if you are unable to do much physically, you can still do a lot emotionally. I may be disabled and it is tough for me to do laundry or even change a light bulb but that has nothing to do with my ability to be valuable as a human being. Just because you are blown out of a lot of activities, doesn't mean you have to stop contributing altogether.

Lynn F.

No one understands just why so many health professionals have been hard-hit by chronic fatigue syndrome, but Lynn F., age fifty-two, is sad testament to this reality. Before illness struck in 1979, she was a registered nurse and the happily married mother of four. When her children reached school age, she enrolled in a master's program, earned her degree—and a promotion to nursing supervisor—and began eyeing a slot as director of nursing. For one shining moment, her career prospects seemed limitless.

Then the world collapsed around her. In the first year of illness, she passed through the revolving door of the hospital more times than she can recall. At first, she was seeking treatment for overwhelming fatigue, stomach and bowel problems, and muscular and joint pain. Doctors could do little for her and eventually she was back in the hospital—this time on the mental health unit being treated for depression. "I had begun to think seriously of suicide," says Lynn, recalling how she once laid out the medication overdose that would transport her beyond the world of pain.

The help of a shrewd psychiatrist pulled her past that bleak phase, but health woes have continued. In 1984, her vocal chords became paralyzed and Lynn could communicate only in a whisper. Terrible sore throats, shortness of breath, and flaring lung problems plagued her. Two years later, balance problems began. Driving a car was already out of the question and then it became impossible for her even to ride in one. Her doctor recommended a wheelchair and Lynn now uses it whenever she anticipates having to walk more than fifty or a hundred feet.

Still the curtain of hope seems to be rising. Recently Lynn and her husband moved from downtown Portland, Oregon, into a ranch-style home in the country. Along with acquiring a spectacular view of Mt. Hood, they can now share a bedroom again. In their old home the master bedroom was on the second floor and Lynn simply couldn't make it up the stairs. An abiding Christian faith, her support group activities, mastery of the art of deep relaxation, and the willingness to accept misfortune have all been sources of strength. "Now when things get bad, I realize I just have to get back in bed," says Lynn.

Nick R.

Slender, with sandy-brown hair and a mischievous glint in his eyes, thirty-five-year-old Nick R. looks like a man with a lot going for him. After a successful career teaching elementary school, he enrolled in a graduate program at the University of Vermont and was aiming for a master's in social work. Then chronic fatigue syndrome mowed him down. "I've been doing battle with this thing since 1985," says Nick R., who speculates that a bout with adult chicken pox a few years earlier might have weakened his resistance. "I don't know what hit me but I began feeling weak and tremendously confused. I was just wiped out."

His symptoms, which he likens to the fog that accompanies sleep deprivation, progressed from bad to worse. "I wouldn't be able to put together a string of words sometimes. Or I'd say things and a minute later not be able to remember what I'd said." Battered by food and mold allergies, especially during the humid New York City summer, Nick began a round of visits to medical experts. He found no satisfaction. "It blew my mind that no doctor would be able to come to an understanding about what was wrong with me," he says.

Ultimately, Nick R. was forced to drop out of school and live on a small inheritance. After doing some of his own research and reading, he radically altered his diet to eliminate highly refined foods and that brought him some relief. The healing powers of time and his willingness to restrict his life-style have also helped, although his ability to concentrate remains weakened and his energy still comes and goes. "A residue of neurological difficulties lingers. I'm still waiting for all the cobwebs to clear," he says.

What are the lessons he has learned from his bout with chronic illness? "I am much more open-minded about life and I've learned not to let small things be bothersome or stressful. I'd like to believe this experience has helped make me a more sensitive person."

Ruth L.

Only one semester before she was to graduate college, Ruth L. came down with infectious mononucleosis. Doctors counseled rest and patience. Eighteen months later, her symptoms were worse than ever and the twenty-year-old political science major was finally diagnosed with chronic fatigue syndrome. Although the label soothed Ruth's worried parents, who had tried to steel themselves against the possibility of a terminal illness, it remains uncertain how long the healing process will take. "It is a wrenching experience to see your child suffer," said Sharon L., Ruth's mother. "She was an 'A' student with a brilliant career ahead of her. Now it seems as though her life is in limbo."

Laboratory tests have identified severe allergies, balance system abnormalities, and a low-grade fever. Ruth L. is too dizzy to drive and suffers from panic attacks that leave her hovering on the edge of control. Stress did not cause her illness, insists the frail student, but it has certainly resulted from it. "The physical problems come first. But when these bizarre things are happening and you don't understand why and you can't control them, it creates emotional problems, too."

The experts think that teenagers and very young adults afflicted with CFS have a particularly difficult time learning to cope because they often lack confidence and a firm sense of themselves. Their peers, who seldom have any firsthand experience with illness or limitations, are likely to look elsewhere for the fun and friendship they crave. Ruth L. concedes that this has happened to her. "Being sick for so long has taken away my dignity and left me feeling humiliated. And my friends simply can't be bothered with someone who is sick. The truth is that unless you have this illness, you just can't understand it."

PART II

The Medical Perspective

2

■

What's Happening to Me? The Course of Chronic Fatigue Syndrome

What is really so extraordinary is that the symptoms constantly change. I'll go through one month of intense body pains and that will be my main problem. The next month it is the intense headaches that overwhelm me. And the month after that, I'll feel physically better but I'll be so panic-stricken that I just want to curl up under the covers and hide.

–Sherry T., age thirty-two, CFS patient,
Atlanta, Georgia

It is the uncertainty that is so difficult to live with. If I knew that I was going to get better in a year, or even five years, I think I could manage. But not to know whether I'll ever be well is devastating.

–Roger P., age twenty-four, CFS patient,
Dallas, Texas

Chronic fatigue syndrome can affect virtually all of the body's major systems: Neurological, immunological, hormonal, gastrointestinal and musculoskeletal problems have been reported. The principle of Murphy's Law—anything that can go wrong will go wrong—could have been written for chronic fatigue syndrome patients, who learn to endure erratic and unpredictable symptoms and an uncertain prognosis.

Chronic fatigue syndrome is a syndrome, meaning a constellation of signs and symptoms, possibly with multiple causes, rather than one discrete disease. The distinction is significant because it helps explain why the course of CFS from onset to recovery varies so much from one patient to another. But regardless of its pattern, the cumulative effect of the ailment's myriad symptoms is the same: to transform ordinary activity into a Herculean challenge. "So much of my day is taken up by things that people take for granted, like cleaning and cooking," says one thirty-eight-year-old woman. "Even the simplest chore has become so much harder. There are times when going to the curb to get the morning's mail is an effort. Dragging myself to the grocery store can consume half a day."

Onset: The Nightmare Begins

The majority of patients can pinpoint the onset of chronic fatigue syndrome to a single day. Characteristically, flu-like symptoms— headache, sore throat, low-grade fever, fatigue, muscle and joint aches—signal the abrupt descent of illness. But initially these symptoms are not cause for great concern. Only when they fail to clear up within a reasonable period of time, or flare into a more acute illness, do patients become alarmed and seek medical help.

Donald S., a forty-one-year-old business writer, has a typical story:

> I can remember the exact day I got sick—January 14, 1985. That morning, I awoke with an achy body, a sore throat, and a temperature that quickly developed into a bad bout of the flu. I took a week off from work, then tried to go back but I just couldn't function. I've been on an extended leave of absence ever since. Frankly, I don't feel as though I ever fully recovered from that first illness. I just never got well.

Some patients remember specific emotional stressors that preceded the sudden onset of sickness. One woman felt the first hints of illness as she returned from her father's funeral and theorizes that the emotional shock sapped her of strength and left her vulnerable to viral invaders. Without recalling a single precipitating crisis, others say that CFS descended during a stressful period of an already stressful life in which job pressures, the strain of juggling career and family, or marital difficulties were taking a psychic toll. But the correlation between stress and chronic fatigue syndrome is often indirect and sometimes nonexistent and most researchers are convinced there are more complex explanations for the eruption of illness.

Sometimes apparently unrelated illnesses or an accident precede CFS. Some patients first have a bout of acute infectious mononucleosis;

indeed the symptoms of mono so closely resemble those of the syndrome that it has been called chronic mononucleosis. A head injury, surgery, or anesthesia are also mentioned as traumas that apparently play a role in triggering illness. Allergic reactions are sometimes involved and a small group of patients feel certain they became ill shortly after using a furniture stripper or another potent household chemical.

Not everyone is flattened overnight. For some, symptoms begin more slowly, insidiously, sapping them of strength and energy over a period of many months. As she reviewed the progression of her disease, Betty P. of Portland, Oregon, recalled: "For more than a year, I thought perhaps I was slightly anemic because I tired more easily than my friends. I often felt achy, too, but I chalked it up to frequent colds and a delicate constitution. With enough rest, I was able to function fairly well." But over the past six months, Betty has noted a marked deterioration. "Gradually the limitations on my energy have worsened. The good days seem to be fewer and fewer and it is getting progressively more difficult to continue working."

Until a cause or causes are identified with certainty, it will be impossible to know just why a stressful event, a seemingly unrelated medical problem, or a particular environmental toxin triggers illness in one person but not in others. Whether the illness of a person who sickens gradually follows a course that is significantly different from someone who is felled in a single swoop also remains unclear. But the similarities and differences in the patterns of onset certainly suggest a number of avenues for research, and in the next chapter we explore the possible causes of CFS and look more closely at current scientific theory.

A Waxing and Waning Pattern

One of the hallmarks of chronic fatigue syndrome is the remarkable fluctuation in the nature and severity of its symptoms. Erratic and unpredictable, they vary from month to month, from day to day, and sometimes from moment to moment. One afternoon a person with CFS may feel energetic and productive and by evening find that severe pain or overwhelming fatigue curtails all activity. Another day improvement may come just as abruptly and just as unexpectedly. "There are times when I can be so ill that my body is just wracked in pain from my head to my toenails and then sometimes out of the blue, it will disappear, leaving me feeling just a little weak," says Marty P. "I will have to pinch myself and say, 'is this really me, could I really have been so sick just half an hour ago?' "

Just as one individual's illness varies from day to day and month to month, so, too, it changes markedly from person to person. Some people have low-grade symptoms all the time; others have periods of remission between episodic illness. One patient may be virtually bedridden for months at a time—an estimated 25 percent of CFS patients are confined to their homes—while others continue working at least part-time but drastically curtail their social and recreational activities. "There is a spectrum of illness with this disease, as with many others," says Dr. Neil Singer. The internist whose practice in the Pacific Heights neighborhood of San Francisco includes hundreds of CFS patients compares the syndrome to a flu virus, noting that both can affect different people in very different ways. Genetic makeup, health history, the availability of medical and social supports, and the prevalence of environmental toxins or allergens all contribute to the relative severity of chronic fatigue syndrome.

Relapse triggers also vary from individual to individual and physicians and patients alike have been frustrated by efforts to understand what makes the illness flare at a particular moment. A marked decline has been observed after too much physical activity, even among people once accustomed to rigorous exercise. Weather changes often take a toll, with some people reacting poorly to the sun and others sensitive to drops or rises in humidity or barometric pressure. Both the wilting heat and humidity of summer and the bitter cold of winter can exacerbate illness. While the causative role of stress stirs controversy, few doubt that it, too, exacerbates symptoms.

A Checklist of Symptoms and Signs

Chronic fatigue syndrome is largely an illness of *symptoms*, rather than *signs*. Medically speaking, a sign is an indicator of illness that can be objectively measured: fever, swollen lymph glands, and weight changes are all signs. A symptom is much more subjective and may have no signs at all associated with it: headaches, fatigue, and soreness are typical symptoms and many others are described below. The burdensome skepticism confronted by so many CFS patients results partly from the fact that neither laboratory tests nor a physical examination can detect the severity of most symptoms.

Symptoms often appear unrelated and sometimes frankly odd.

"For a while I had the most agonizing toothache. I went to the dentist and told him I couldn't bear it, he should just pull all of my teeth out. But he couldn't find anything wrong with my teeth and after a couple of weeks the pain vanished," said one woman in exasperation. Another reports a "creepy crawler sensation" in which she felt as though her skin had spiders crawling all over it, again a symptom for which no medical explanation could be found. Physicians who treat CFS with any regularity say they are no longer surprised by patient complaints. "At first, these symptoms seemed bizarre to me," said San Francisco Bay area physician Carol Jessop. "Now they are as familiar as the back of my hand."

Dr. Stephen E. Straus, a leading CFS researcher at the National Institute of Allergy and Infectious Diseases (NIAID), a branch of the National Institutes of Health, summarizes the symptoms and signs reported by his patients as follows:

Easy fatigability	100 percent
Difficulty concentrating	90
Headache	90
Sore throat	85
Tender lymph nodes	80
Muscle aches	80
Joint aches	75
Feverishness	75
Difficulty sleeping	70
Psychiatric problems	65
Allergies	55
Abdominal cramps	40
Weight loss	20
Rash	10
Rapid pulse	10
Weight gain	5
Chest pain	5
Night sweat	5

Source: "The Chronic Mononucleosis Syndrome," *Journal of Infectious Diseases*, March 1988.

Other physicians and many of the patient support groups around the country add scores of other symptoms and signs to this list, including:

- Balance disorders
- Phobias and anxiety
- Mood swings
- Ringing in the ears
- Seeing spots
- Disorientation
- Memory loss
- Inability to focus attention
- Difficulty pronouncing or remembering words
- Inability to do simple math problems
- Irregular heartbeat
- Frequent respiratory tract infections
- Nausea
- Diarrhea, constipation, or both
- Frequent or uncomfortable urination
- Frequent urinary tract or vaginal yeast infections
- Prostate pain
- Sensitivity to sunlight
- Alcohol or caffeine intolerance
- Menstrual cycle changes
- Thyroid inflammation
- Bleeding gums, mouth sores
- Swelling of feet, face, hands
- Chills or body temperature below normal
- Nightmares
- Awakening with a hung-over feeling, despite sufficient sleep
- Back pain over the kidneys

While any or all of these symptoms and signs can herald chronic fatigue syndrome, they can also warn of other medical problems. Extreme caution must be taken to avoid stumbling into the easy trap of attributing any new medical development to CFS. Whether a disease that is more treatable or one that poses graver risks is presenting itself, patients and physicians have a shared responsibility for remaining alert to any harbinger of change.

Overpowering Fatigue

Fatigue is one of the most common symptoms reported to family-care physicians and it can accompany a wide range of diseases, from the common cold to cancer. But clinicians say there is a clear distinction between ordinary fatigue and the exhaustion that is the hallmark of CFS. "I hear complaints from people who are tired all day long but it is just not the same sort of devastating fatigue. I had never heard of this except in patients who are preterminal," says Dr. Jessop, who argues that a more appropriate name for the illness is "devastating fatigue syndrome."

While there are really no words adequate to the task of describing the incapacitating fatigue endured by CFS patients, their own voices say it best:

- "It feels as though someone pulled a plug out on you. This has just drained every ounce of my energy."

- "This is not ordinary exhaustion. After a night's sleep, I awaken feeling as though I have just finished a ten-mile run. When I stand up, it is as if I am carrying someone else on my shoulders."

- I have sat at dinner in a restaurant and by the time the main course is finished, I feel that I have to lay down on the floor. It is a crushing sort of fatigue. You just cannot rally the forces to care about anything."

- "I had no strength at all. If I got up in the middle of the night, often I would have to crawl back to bed. Getting up and taking a shower in the morning felt like a hard day's work."

- "People always ask, 'what did you do over the weekend,' and they expect to hear you went to the movies or out to dinner. No one wants to hear that I spent the entire weekend in bed."

• "I would lie for hours and hours watching the squirrels move
back and forth. To fix lunch would take about four trips to the
kitchen. I'd put the kettle on for tea, then flop back into bed
for a rest. Then I'd get the bread out and flop again. Finally I'd
return to make the sandwich, and on my last trip, I might be
able to sit down and have lunch."

A complaint of fatigue is known in medical parlance as a "soft"
finding because it cannot be formally measured with a laboratory test
or physical exam. It is also nonspecific, meaning that no precise
diagnosis can be derived from the symptom. But to individuals who
lose the verve that once animated their lives, the paralyzing consequences of fatigue are both real and cataclysmic.

Sleep Disorders

Sleep patterns of chronic fatigue syndrome sufferers are typically dis-
turbed. Despite bone-tired exhaustion and a craving for deep, uninter-
rupted sleep, it is rare for patients to awaken in the morning feeling
well-rested. Disorders associated with CFS take different forms. Some
people suffer severe insomnia, tossing and turning for hours at a time.
Others sleep a few hours and then bolt awake, feeling wired and
unable to return to unconsciousness.

Most common of all is the inability to obtain consistent rapid-eye
movement sleep (REM), which is considered crucial to a good night's
rest. Occupying about 20 percent of an average night's sleep, REM is
the excitable stage, when heart rate and blood pressure alternately
shoot up, then plunge back down, blood flow to the brain increases,
and dreams are vivid. When a person sleeps fitfully, rapidly alternat-
ing between light sleep, REM sleep, and wakefulness, it is almost
impossible to feel sufficiently rested.

The relationship between sleep problems and poor health is cyclical.
CFS-linked pain, depression, and anxiety interfere with good sleep,
which in turn exacerbates symptoms of pain, depression, and anxiety.
Although certain medications can improve the quality of sleep, others
disrupt it, so your doctors should be aware of your sleep troubles.

Depression

Although no one fully understands the link between the two conditions, depression and chronic fatigue syndrome are often tightly inter-

woven. But the symptoms of CFS do not fit the description of *exogenous* depression, which is a well-understood mental illness in which external factors provoke depression. Nor is there consistent evidence of recent trauma or the personal or family history among patients that would lend support to a diagnosis of primary depression.

Rather, CFS-related depression appears to be *endogenous* in nature, meaning that it has physiological origins within the body. "I don't even like to use the term depression because it implies that you can just snap out of this," says Dr. Edwin A. Jacobson, a Beverly Hills internist with a particular interest in treating CFS patients. "It is important to educate both physicians and patients that this is a different form of depression. It's not something patients have control over, it's not something they did to themselves and they can't wish it away."

Unfortunately, secondary depression, which follows from disease, rather than causes it, is as hard to measure and just as disabling as a psychiatric disorder. Nonetheless, the distinction has important implications for treatment—simply knowing that there is a chemical basis for your mood swings and that they are directly related to illness can be tremendously reassuring.

Vestibular Disorders

Disorders of the balance, or vestibular, system are very common among CFS sufferers. Modulated by the inner ear, our system of balance is more vulnerable than many people realize. Infections, traumas, any event that causes chemical changes in the brain, from emotional stress to pregnancy, and even prolonged or turbulent air travel can throw it out of kilter. Depending on its cause, a balance disorder may occur continually or recur periodically. Changes in altitude or barometric pressure sometimes provoke problems and so can a quick change of head position in susceptible individuals.

Balance disorders most often manifest themselves in the form of lightheadedness, dizziness, vertigo, or nausea. The Vestibular Disorders Association of America describes severe balance problems as "a prolonged period of violent, whirling sensations where the world is spinning out of control." Bright wall colors or wild-patterned rugs can be inordinately distracting to CFS patients, making concentration impossible. Words may appear to jump all over the printed page and patients also report an incessant ringing in their ears (tinnitus). Walking is sometimes difficult, with patients tilting off balance or stumbling to the ground for no apparent reason.

Irrational phobias, especially in patients who have never experienced them before, can be related to balance disorders. One CFS patient likened an anxiety attack to the instant just before a fall: "Think of that feeling you get in the pit of your stomach when you are sure something horrible is about to happen. Imagine trying to function with that sensation all the time," said Sandy, a thirty-five-year-old woman whose balance-related phobias have kept her virtually housebound.

Cognitive Dysfunction

In a moving plea for compassion and effective treatment, one young patient provided a long list of the incapacitating physical discomforts that he now endures, then added, "But what I miss most is my mind."

Perhaps the most bizarre of the symptoms that accompany chronic fatigue syndrome are cognition problems. Berkeley psychologists Dr. Sheila Bastien and Dr. Robert S. Thomas, who have conducted neuropsychological assessments of more than 150 CFS patients, report finding significant impairments in memory, concentration, and spatial and motor functioning in many of them. More severely ill patients demonstrate problems with verbal fluency, response time, and the abilities to perform calculations and to reason abstractly. One man says his confusion evokes the fuzziness of a hangover and recalls:

> I would be unable to remember a conversation I had ten minutes ago. I'd lose my keys and go into a panic attack because I had no idea where they could be. Sounds trivial but imagine having it happen five times during the course of a day. On more than one occasion I'd be driving and suddenly be totally unable to remember where I was going.

Other incidents that clearly point to impaired mental capacities would be humorous were they not so poignant. A woman in Charlotte, North Carolina, recalled that she was once totally unable to remember her own telephone number, although she had lived in the same house for fourteen years. Out of desperation, she finally called directory assistance and when the operator recited the number, it didn't sound the least bit familiar. The husband of another patient explains that he no longer asks his wife for directions because she is likely to say, "hang a reft," then look perplexed when no one understands her meaning.

Exercise Exhaustion

One of the hallmarks of chronic fatigue syndrome is an inability to tolerate exercise. Typically, a patient who maintained a vigorous exercise regimen before falling ill now feels exhausted after climbing a flight of stairs. The man who jogged six miles a day finds it an effort to walk five blocks to the corner grocery store. The swimmer who swam lap after lap suffers a bout of chills and fever each time she approaches a pool. Just why exercise aggravates the symptoms of CFS remains a mystery but the pattern is so characteristic that some physicians consider it an important diagnostic hint.

The Prognosis: Will I Ever Be Well?

Whatever their particular symptoms, chronic fatigue syndrome patients share at least one characteristic in common: the sense of having been deprived of all they have striven to accomplish and much of what they have earned. One woman recalls that when she was awarded her master's degree in public administration, her mother told her with pride that nothing could ever take away that education. Now, she notes mournfully, "I feel that my education *has* been taken away from me. I don't know whether I will ever be able to put it to use."

Despite all the unknowns and uncertainties surrounding the enigma of chronic fatigue syndrome, patients can be reassured that the illness is seldom progressive and is assuredly not fatal. No objective evidence—such as drastically worsening laboratory test results—suggests a precipitous decline in health. And many patients do recover, some within the first year or two of illness, others after many years of erratic symptoms. Dr. Anthony Komaroff, the researcher associated with Brigham and Women's Hospital in Boston, estimates that the average duration of illness is 2.9 years, with a range between 6 months and 13 years. Many physicians have noted that if patients are going to have a downward course, it happens in the first year or two of illness. Afterward their condition tends to stabilize, although functional level is often reduced. Says Dr. Carol Jessop:

> People accommodate their lives to this illness. They get used to the quirky kinds of things that happen and to not having the same kind of energy they once did. They become grateful when they have a day with 50 percent of their previous energy rather than just 10 percent of their energy, whereas before 50 percent was terribly upsetting to them.

Since CFS has not been closely tracked for very long, statistics on recovery and susceptibility to relapse are not terribly reliable. But anecdotal evidence is hopeful. "I feel infinitely better," says thirty-five-year-old Nick R. of Queens, New York, whose activities were severely restricted for almost three years. "My energy still comes and goes and in the summer my allergies flare and some of the symptoms return. But my main concern now is how to plug back into the work world. My self-esteem has really taken a battering but I'm feeling optimistic again. And I sense myself getting stronger all the time."

Recovery often comes so slowly that it can only be measured by comparing one's present physical limitations with those of a year or two before. Patients may still tire more easily than in the past and are advised to take precautions to maintain their improved health status; commonsense measures such as eating well, reducing stress, and resting whenever necessary can make an enormous difference. Even patients far along the road to recovery suffer periodic bad spells, but these are less severe and shorter-lived than in the past and generally they bounce back to good health more quickly than before.

Alas, once burned, twice scarred, and no man or woman who has been felled by CFS ever rests entirely easy. As the illness goes into remission, fears linger that it may return uninvited, unannounced, and most certainly unwelcome. "None of us trust our health any more," says Bob Landau, the New Jersey support group leader. It will require many years of patient follow-up studies to know just how valid those fears really are.

Some Commonly Asked Questions

Am I Contagious?

One of the questions asked most fearfully by CFS patients is, "Am I contagious?" We won't know the answer with certainty until we identify the culprit in the illness, but a full-blown case of chronic fatigue syndrome is not likely to be casually transmitted.

An important reason why is that most of the viral suspects in CFS—notably those in the herpes family—are already quite common in this country. Thus the majority of the adult population has already developed antibodies to them; most of the remaining population can easily do so upon first exposure. And individuals who cannot effectively resist infection cannot do much about avoiding exposure because so many common viruses are shed periodically through an infected person's saliva. Speaking about HHV6, the most recently discovered herpes virus, Dr. Paul Cheney said, "Radical alterations of life-style to avoid it are silly. There's not an island remote enough or a hole deep enough that will allow you to hide from a herpes virus."

Even if a contagious virus is implicated in CFS, less easily transmissible factors are almost certainly involved as well. Environmental pollutants, stress, and immune system irregularities, all of which have been mentioned as cofactors in the syndrome, are certainly not contagious. And there have been relatively few cases in which friends, lovers, or roommates appear to have "caught" the illness from one another. Where illness has spread within a family, it usually moves from parent to child, or between brother and sister, supporting the relevance of genetic predisposition. Nonetheless, there are certain commonsense precautions recommended for CFS patients and anyone close to them. The uncertainties surrounding the illness make it advisable that CFS patients not donate blood. If other members of your family have been diagnosed with the syndrome and you are seized with similar symptoms, be certain to keep your physician fully informed. Finally, talk candidly to your partner. Unless the channels of communication are kept wide open, a lover is almost certain to harbor secret fears of falling ill. One woman complained to her doctor: "My husband hasn't touched me in seven months. He thinks he can catch CFS in the same way you can catch AIDS." This type of misinformation can destroy a relationship far more quickly than chronic fatigue syndrome itself.

Am I at Higher Risk for Other Diseases?

The long-run implications of chronic fatigue syndrome simply aren't known yet because the illness has been under close scrutiny for such a short period of time. But there is cause for optimism. CFS patients have not been plagued by the opportunistic infections that batter persons with AIDS nor have they reported a rash of unrelated sickness.

A wave of panic washed over patients when rumors spread of a scientific study that linked CFS and cancer. A closer reading of the study, published by Dr. James Jones of the National Jewish Center for Immunology and Respiratory Medicine in the March 24, 1988, edition of *New England Journal of Medicine,* actually suggests no such thing. Although Dr. Jones did report three cases of a rare cancer in patients who also exhibited many of the signs and symptoms common to CFS, he emphasized that the cases were noteworthy simply because they were so unique. The distinctive feature of his findings was that the Epstein-Barr virus, previously thought to attack only the antibody-producing B cells of the immune system, had caused a T-cell cancer (these and other components of the immune system are explained in the next chapter). Dr. Jones said: "I had an obligation to advise the scientific community that the spectrum of EBV disease is broader than previously expected. But I don't want physicians or patients with Epstein-Barr virus infections to try to draw a connection. There isn't any."

The possibility of an increased risk of cancer among CFS patients cannot be entirely dismissed, however. In a small study of a cluster outbreak in a symphony orchestra, Dr. Seymour Grufferman of the Pittsburgh Cancer Institute concluded the cancer threat was real and other researchers have suggested a depressed immune system could allow cancerous cells to replicate. More research is clearly needed in this key area.

Can I Get Pregnant?

The simple answer is yes, absolutely. There is no medical reason that a woman with chronic fatigue syndrome cannot become pregnant and safely carry a baby to term. Often women actually improve during pregnancy and there is no evidence that their babies are at increased risk of congenital abnormalities or jaundice. Some researchers believe that women with CFS are slightly more likely to miscarry or to give birth to a low-weight baby but the data here are not definitive. Unlike AIDS, chronic fatigue syndrome apparently cannot be passed from mother to her fetus or newborn infant.

Unfortunately there are other practical considerations to bear in mind. At age thirty-eight, JoAnna S. of Seattle is acutely aware that her biological clock is ticking. Her fervent wish to have children has been held in abeyance for three years as she struggles against the exhausting effects of chronic fatigue syndrome. She wonders now whether the opportunity will ever come.

> I would love to get pregnant but I'm just now starting to feel a little better and I don't think I'd have the strength to cope with a difficult pregnancy. And I worry about being able to give my child proper attention. Children demand so much energy and my physical resources are still so limited.

JoAnna's concerns are legitimate but other women report the picture is not uniformly bleak. Sara B., age thirty-one, who became ill shortly after the birth of her first child, says she has no regrets. Caring for Heather has not been easy, she'll admit, but crucial support from her husband and parents has made it possible. The two-year-old girl is 100 percent healthy, and Sara says: "My energy level for dealing with her comes in waves. But she gets all the attention I can give—I've really changed my priorities and the sacrifice has been well worth it. I can't imagine life without Heather."

Physicians express somewhat more concern about women who develop chronic fatigue syndrome during their pregnancy. Very little research has been done in this area but it is known that the risk to a fetus is heightened with any viral illness, particularly in a woman's first trimester. Until specific viruses are positively identified in chronic fatigue syndrome and research studies are undertaken, however, undue alarm is pointless.

Is There Any Connection Between CFS and AIDS?

The acquired immune deficiency syndrome (AIDS) leaves its victims susceptible to brutal opportunistic infections, is progressive, and thus far, is invariably fatal. Chronic fatigue syndrome is none of these things. No credible arguments have been made to link AIDS to CFS and comparisons between the two only reflect fear and often ignorance—and yet they surface time and time again. "No matter what I tell my neighbors, they think I have AIDS," says one CFS patient.

The reason is clear. AIDS has brought far more than personal tragedy to its unlucky victims. It has also introduced a sense of vulnerability to a generation that harbors no memories of an epidemic since polio and that has taken its good health for granted. For the first time in most of our lives, we have watched our peers endure a lingering illness and die a painful death. Many of us have borne witness to the devastating vulnerability of a human being whose immune system has malfunctioned. We now know that an onslaught of vicious viruses, parasites, and bacteria can mount an attack on a body that lacks the resources to fight back.

With AIDS so fresh in our minds, it is frightening to think that chronic fatigue syndrome may be linked to a damaged immune system. Unfortunately, there is some indication of immune system abnormalities in the bodies of chronic fatigue syndrome patients and the effort to understand them is a critical direction of current research. But in marked contrast to AIDS, persons with CFS do not become progressively sicker, they are not susceptible to worsening infection, and in time, many of them do recover.

The next chapter looks more closely at the evidence of immunological irregularities and attempts to develop a coherent theory about the cause of chronic fatigue syndrome. It also considers a possible role for viruses, allergies, stress, and environmental toxins.

3

■

On the Trail
of the Culprit:
Speculations on Cause

Does the syndrome exist? Absolutely. But the question is, is it a single entity, and the odds are it probably is not. Is it caused by a single factor? Most certainly not. There are lots of hypotheses about the syndrome, all of which are open to examination and consideration.

–Dr. Stephen E. Straus,
National Institute of Allergy and Infectious Disease,
Bethesda, Maryland

Only two facts can be categorically stated about the cause of chronic fatigue syndrome: No one knows and speculations abound. One physician declares with undocumented certainty, "there is no viral component to this syndrome" while another insists "it is assuredly a viral disease with a psychological overlay." Researchers cite evidence of immune system abnormalities but report inconsistent findings. Some think increased environmental toxins have damaged our health, while others argue that emotional pressures are literally making people sick.

Other, more speculative, theories abound. Two researchers have independently suggested that the widespread use of vaccinations, notably a new rubella vaccine introduced in the late 1970s, is at fault. The implication here is that tinkering with antibody-producing cells has backfired, weakening the immune system. A link between CFS and candidiasis, or yeast toxins, has also been proposed.

45

The true cause may be a complex interrelationship among all these factors, some of them, or none at all. "I doubt any one thing causes it," says Dr. Edwin Jacobson, the Beverly Hills internist. "I think it is a combination of things that all come together in a susceptible person." Dr. Steven Marlowe, an infectious disease specialist in Atlanta, Georgia, confirms that perspective: "I think there are multiple causes. My guess is that chronic fatigue syndrome is the final common pathway for a variety of infectious and perhaps noninfectious agents."

Exactly which viral agents, how much stress, and which environmental poisons are involved remains to be determined, as does the relative importance of each factor and the reason that certain individuals become ill while others do not. Improper functioning of the immune system also appears to play a role in the illness but we don't yet know whether it is a cause or an effect. If CFS has viral origins, for example, why does the immune system fail to marshall its forces against an invader? One theory suggests that certain individuals have a genetic weakness that renders them incapable of resisting a particular virus. Or a cyclical process may be involved in which some combination of viral invaders, stress, and environmental toxins weaken the immune system, leaving it vulnerable to further attack.

On the frontiers of medical research, scientists are devoting substantial energy to a unifying hypothesis that may pinpoint the cause of chronic fatigue syndrome. Broadly, the hypothesis suggests that CFS begins when an inciting agent—most likely a virus, possibly a bacteria or an allergen—triggers an initially normal immune system response. Rather than return to its quiescent state once the invader is subdued, however, the immune system continues instead to produce the potent substances that cause many of the disabling symptoms of CFS. In this grand unification theory, the immune system is not simply overactive. Components of it are also underactive— weakened perhaps by stress, environmental toxins, or genetic deficits—so that immune response to further infectious agents is sluggish.

Honing in on the cause of chronic fatigue syndrome is a key scientific priority. Until we fully understand why the illness takes root, we cannot effectively treat it, cure it, or halt its relentless march through our society.

The Human Immune System:
A Defending Army

A brief look at how a well-tooled immune system protects the body from illness is crucial to understanding the factors that might cause chronic fatigue syndrome.

The millions of white blood cells born in the bone marrow lie at the heart of an astonishingly complex and effective defense system. Three types of white blood cells—phagocytes and two classes of lymphocytes, the T cells and the B cells, each with several subsets—work in tandem to neutralize or destroy a foreign invader, be it a virus, bacteria, fungus, parasite, or a portion of these organisms, before it can damage the body.

The *phagocytes* are the immune system's first line of defense. Constantly prowling through the bloodstream on the lookout for signs of an enemy, phagocytes are programmed to engulf and digest micro-organisms, pollutants, dust particles, or cellular debris that do not belong in the body. When the foreign invader is a virus, the *macrophage* class of phagocytes plucks a protein particle from the invader and displays it on its cellular surface like a prize of war.

Now the macrophage must literally bump into the *helper T cells* specifically programmed to combat the viral *antigen*. When they meet, the macrophage secretes *interleukin-1*, a protein that commands those specifically matched helper T cells to replicate. As they multiply, the helper T cells, in turn, secrete *lymphokines*, potent chemicals manufactured in the lymph nodes that include *interferons*, a family of antiviral proteins, and other interleukins. These lymphokines stimulate the production of more macrophages as well as *B cells* and *killer T cells*.

The B cells multiply and then begin to manufacture *antibodies*, potent chemical weapons designed to neutralize and counteract anti-gens. Antibodies are manufactured to combat specific antigens, much as a key is designed to fit just one lock. They are grouped into one of five major categories of *immunoglobulin* molecules: IgM antibodies generally appear early in an immune response; IgG, the most common immunoglobulin, appear later; IgA antibodies predominate in the gastrointestinal and respiratory tracts and in secretions, such as saliva and tears; IgE antibodies trigger certain allergic responses; IgD, the fifth major category of immunoglobulins is not yet well understood.

Antibodies perform a number of different functions: Sometimes they actually kill invaders; they can also make them more attractive

targets for phagocytes to devour and they can block viruses from
penetrating human cells to wreak further damage. It is not enough,
however, to kill the viruses circulating through the bloodstream. The
immune system must also have a way to disrupt the viral replication
process taking place within the human cells. Enter the *natural killer
(NK) cells* and *killer T cells*.

Natural killer cells are not programmed to respond only to
specific antigens. Instead they are on the front lines of attack, keeping
the body under constant surveillance in order to disintegrate any
tumor or virus-infected cells they encounter. The killer cells of the
immune system work in one of two ways: First, they can puncture the
cells, forcing the release of their contaminated contents and enabling
other components of the immune system to handle the remnants; or
they can precipitate a chemical reaction that destroys infected cells
directly. The genius of these aggressors is that they sacrifice only
infected cells, usually leaving others unscathed.

After an attack against an invader has been successful, the *suppressor T cells* call off the immune system response, deactivating other T
and B cells and returning the body to equilibrium. Memory B and T
cells continue to circulate through the bloodstream, vigilant against
the return of the same virus. If an infection reoccurs, memory cells
enable the immune system to rev up its attack more quickly.

Where the Immune System
Can Go Wrong

Although it is a finely tuned work of evolutionary art, a great many
factors can interfere with the proper functioning of the immune
system. Advancing age, previous illness, stress, and environmental
toxins can all depress its ability to combat foreign invaders. When a
virus specifically targets the cells of the immune system—as with
AIDS, which disarms the T cells—the functional capacity of the
immune system is also severely compromised.

A number of scientific papers have found evidence of immunologic alterations in CFS patients, although the findings have not
been consistent enough to be definitive. Still, in the era of AIDS any
suggestion that the immune system has gone awry is frightening.
Therefore, it is important to remember that subtle alterations of the
body's most important protective mechanism in no way suggests that
it is on the brink of complete collapse. Nor is there any evidence

whatsoever that once altered slightly, the immune system is likely to degenerate progressively. Dr. Stephen Straus of the National Institute of Allergy and Infectious Disease is quite emphatic on this point:

> There is a common notion that the immune system represents some kind of delicate balance and you have to sit at this central point and be maintained there. If you teeter a little bit to the side, you are going to roll down the hill and fall off, that it is going to progress.
>
> The fact is that the immune system cannot be constructed that way because it has to constantly handle insults, has to constantly accept challenges that gets it off center. And it has to have some ways of coming back. My suspicion is that the immune system can tolerate pretty well a fair range of differences.

An Overactive Immune System?

One theory receiving particularly close scrutiny from researchers at the National Institutes of Health is the role of *cytokines* in chronic fatigue syndrome. Cytokines are naturally occurring substances released by human cells during infection in order to regulate the immune response. Lymphokines and macrophage-secreted interleukin-1, described earlier in this chapter, are both cytokines.

Although the production of interleukins and interferons is part of a healthy immune system response, it can actually cause some of the symptoms that are common among CFS patients. Interleukin-1, for example, has been shown to produce the fever that often accompanies flu-like illness. One research study showed that cancer patients treated with interleukin-2, a protein used to regulate immune response, suffered some of the neuropsychiatric side effects that are so striking in CFS. Severe lethargy, muscle aches, and memory problems were among the identified side effects. And when monkeys were given interferon, their brain-wave pattern closely resembled that of people who have been diagnosed with depression.

The discomfort associated with these cytokines is a signal that the body is fighting infection and it is often a necessary part of the healing process. In the immune system of a healthy individual, cytokine production is halted once the infection is controlled. Body temperature then returns to normal, and flu-like symptoms disappear.

Scientists speculate about the production of cytokines continuing unchecked in CFS patients. If so, an individual would almost certainly continue to feel the fatigue, muscle aches, malaise, and other symptoms associated with flu-like illness. Preliminary research lends credibility to this theory and it is one of the most promising current avenues of investigation.

An Autoimmune Disorder?

The theory that chronic fatigue syndrome patients suffer from an overactive immune system fits neatly with the notion that CFS is an autoimmune disorder. An autoimmune disorder occurs when the immune system's recognition apparatus goes awry, allowing it to confuse body cells or organs with the foreign invaders it is trained to attack. In response to a wrongly perceived danger, the body manufactures antibodies against itself, known as autoantibodies, and launches an inappropriate onslaught against the body's own parts. The exact cause of most common autoimmune disorders, which include systemic lupus erythematosus (commonly known as lupus), multiple sclerosis, rheumatoid arthritis, and thyroiditis, is poorly understood.

The hypothesis that CFS is also an autoimmune disorder is unproven but there is suggestive circumstantial evidence to support it. For one thing, the patient profiles are similar: Typically women are more susceptible than men and most often become ill between the ages of twenty and forty. Some of the symptoms of chronic fatigue syndrome so closely resemble those of an autoimmune illness that CFS has frequently been mistaken for both multiple sclerosis and lupus. In addition, a family history of autoimmune disease is fairly common among chronic fatigue syndrome patients, which clearly suggests some sort of genetic link.

The Role of Allergies

According to Denver researcher Dr. James Jones, some 50 to 80 percent of all CFS patients suffer from allergies, a marked contrast with the 17 percent of the general American population. A history of allergies predated the illness of some chronic fatigue patients; others developed severe allergies after falling ill. Regardless of onset, many CFS patients now say that their symptoms noticeably worsen during allergy season or whenever they are exposed to a known allergen.

An allergic reaction occurs when the body mistakenly identifies a harmless substance—such as pollen, cat hairs, or house dust—as a foreign invader and musters the full defenses of the immune system in response. This is known as an IgE-mediated allergy, named after the class of antibodies that is produced to combat the allergen. When an allergen collides with an IgE antibody, histamine and other chemicals are released by the cells. Histamine causes many of the familiar allergy symptoms, including watery eyes, sneezing, and a runny nose.

While the precise connection between allergies and chronic fatigue syndrome is murky, the link offers a clue to the distinctive immunological features that have been identified in CFS patients. Researchers speculate that the same mechanism that triggers an overly energetic immune system response to allergens may also account for the inappropriate vigor with which the body responds to other challenges, such as a viral infection.

Some allergists also contend that sensitivities to food, notably yeast products, and a variety of substances in the environment—including petrochemicals, chlorine, sulfur, and ammonia—can cause serious health problems. Clinical ecology or environmental medicine, as the field is known, represents a burgeoning but unorthodox area of study that could have implications for chronic fatigue syndrome patients. Environmental factors are discussed in greater detail later in this chapter.

Other Immunological Abnormalities

A number of important studies lend credibility to speculation that chronic fatigue syndrome results at least in part from immune system abnormalities. In June 1991, four Miami researchers published the results of a thirty patient study in the *Journal of Clinical Microbiology* in which they found a consistent pattern of multiple irregularities. Ongoing work in this groundbreaking field is fueling hope for new insights.

Transforming B Cells. Ground-breaking research at the National Jewish Center for Immunology and Respiratory Medicine has shown that B-cell transformation occurs in about one-third of CFS patients. Cell transformation occurs when a virus infects a cell after which the viral DNA sometimes becomes incorporated into the cellular DNA. DNA is a nucleic acid genetically encoded to enable a cell to make exact copies of itself. Viral infiltration thus alters the reproduction process of the human cell. Although we don't know precisely how this relates to disease process, we do know that a comparable finding is rare in healthy people.

Natural Killer Cells. In November 1987, the prestigious *Journal of Immunology* reported that chronic fatigue syndrome patients exhibit an abnormally low level of natural killer cells, a finding that has since been confirmed by other researchers. The deficiency was pinpointed to an NK-cell subset NKH 1^+T3^-, ordinarily the most populous of the natural killer subsets. Because NK cells are trained to destroy virus-contaminated cells, scientists speculate that deficiencies might leave the body more susceptible to disease. A great deal more research remains to be done in this arena but scientists consider it a major breakthrough.

Helper/Suppressor T-Cell Ratios. Researchers studying the epidemic in Incline Village, Nevada, observed that the helper:suppressor T-cell ratio was unusually high in many patients, apparently reflecting a drop in normal suppressor T cells. Since the suppressor T cells are charged with the mission of restoring equilibrium to the immune system, this finding supports the theory that the immune system fails to disengage after subduing a foreign invader.

Circulating Immune Complexes. According to the National Institutes of Health, about one-third of CFS patients have shown slightly high levels of circulating immune complexes, which are large molecules formed when an antigen and an antibody bind together. High levels of immune complex are often involved in autoimmune diseases and can cause acute inflammation and other symptoms.

Suppressed Immunoglobulin Secretions. A number of CFS patients secrete below-normal levels of several categories of immunoglobulins, notably the IgA molecules, which are bacterial or viral antibodies generally found in secretions and in the respiratory and gastrointestinal tracts. Possibly these suppressed secretions dispose some individuals to a variety of infectious diseases.

Cell-mediated Immunity. Although medical journal reports are few, some doctors have observed a reduced or absent cell-mediated immune (CMI) response in CFS patients. The CMI response, which involves the T lymphocytes, is crucial to the body's capacity to fight certain infectious agents and is commonly absent or lessened in patients with immune deficiency disorders, infections, cancer and autoimmune disease.

The Enigmatic Virus

The word *virus* comes from the Latin for a slimy liquid, stench, or poison, an appropriate derivation for a submicroscopic organism that reproduces by invading human cells and redirecting cellular functions toward its own ends. Unlike all species of plants, animals, and even bacteria, which contain both DNA and RNA—known as the building blocks of life—viruses contain only one or the other. Outside of cells, viruses are little more than inert specks of protein-coated genetic material, incapable of feeding themselves, growing, or replicating.

The evil genius of a virus derives from its capacity to hijack living cells and to force them to do its bidding. At least 300 known viruses in seventeen different family groupings can infect human cells. Once a virus penetrates the membrane of a cell, it can remain latent inside its unsuspecting host for months, even years. Or it may quickly release its RNA or DNA strand and trick the cell into reading the genetic instructions to create carbon copies of the virus.

Newly replicated viruses then escape, sometimes leaving the host cell essentially unscathed, and drift through the bloodstream until they commandeer other cells. But they can also lyse a cell, forcing the invaded host to burst open and die in order to release the newly replicated viruses. A virus may also transform a cell so that each time the host cell reproduces itself, the virus within the cell is reproduced as well. A transforming virus is an ideal candidate for recurring infection.

It now seems likely that chronic fatigue syndrome is not caused by a single virus; possibly, however, the synergistic effect of two or more viruses plays a role in the illness; or CFS patients may share an abnormal immunologic response to viruses in general. If so, the specific virus involved is less significant than the fact that the body's immune system is unable to subdue it. This theory jibes neatly with the concept of an overactive immune system and is supported by the fact that many patients exhibit abnormally high antibody levels to a number of viruses, notably several of the herpes viruses.

Herpes Viruses

Three of the six known herpes viruses are receiving close attention in CFS research: Epstein-Barr, human herpes virus-6 (HHV6) and cytomegalovirus (CMV). The others—herpes simplex I and II, which cause oral and genital herpes, respectively, and zoster varicella, which causes chicken pox and shingles, a painful nerve disease—have not been directly implicated as causative factors, although some patients cannot readily control any herpes infection.

Once infected, human beings carry herpes viruses in the body for life. Ordinarily the immune system keeps them in check but when immune function is compromised—as when an individual is under stress, suffering from unrelated illness, or taking certain types of medication—latent viruses can be prodded into an attack.

Epstein-Barr Virus (EBV). The most renowned viral suspect in chronic fatigue syndrome is the Epstein-Barr virus. Best known as the cause of infectious mononucleosis, the "kissing disease" of adolescence, Epstein-Barr is a transforming virus that has also been implicated in several types of cancer, including nasopharyngeal carcinoma, Burkitt's lymphoma, and other B-cell lymphomas. Those malignancies are relatively rare, however: Some 90 percent of the American population has been infected with EBV by the age of thirty and most of us, of course, show no sign of illness.

In 1985, when researchers first suggested a link between active EBV infection and chronic, unexplained illness, the ailment was called Chronic Epstein-Barr Virus Syndrome, or CEBV. Now, however, it is clear that the syndrome's cause cannot be so simply explained. Although many adults with chronic fatigue syndrome do have elevated EBV antibody levels, others do not. Conversely, signs of EBV antibodies appear in a significant number of healthy people. And some patients with elevated titers (levels of antibodies) to Epstein-Barr virus also have high antibody levels to many other viruses, suggesting that the activation of EBV is a symptom of illness, rather than its cause. Researchers haven't abandoned their interest in the Epstein-Barr virus, however, and the search for a pattern to EBV antibody levels in chronic fatigue syndrome patients continues.

Human Herpesvirus-6 (HHV6). In 1986, Dr. Robert C. Gallo, the National Cancer Institute scientist credited with identifying the AIDS virus, and top researcher S. Zaki Salahuddin heralded the discovery of a previously unknown herpes virus. Human B-cell lymphotropic virus (HBLV) or human herpesvirus-6 (HHV6) became the first herpes virus to be identified since M. A. Epstein and Y. M. Barr reported on the existence of the Epstein-Barr virus in 1964. The discovery of HHV6 was directly linked to ongoing AIDS research: The virulent virus was first isolated in AIDS patients whose depressed immune systems have provided an extraordinary research laboratory.

Although it is not new, HHV6 quickly became a suspect in chronic fatigue syndrome. HHV6 targets both the B and the T cells of the immune system and researchers have speculated that the viral invader might upset the delicate balance between the Epstein-Barr virus and the immune system, awakening EBV from its latent state.

In tests of some 300 CFS patients from Incline Village, Boston, Bethesda, and elsewhere, National Institutes of Health researchers found HHV6 antibodies, indicating a latent or active infection, more than 80 percent of the time. By contrast, only 35 to 45 percent of control populations in those areas had positive HHV6 antibody tests. However, many scientists think that infection rates in the general population will prove to be much higher—possibly matching the prevalence of the Epstein Barr virus—as more sophisticated blood tests are developed. Thus, the significance of the 80 percent figure remains unclear.

HHV6 itself poses serious challenges to researchers attempting to study it because it is so destructive. A lysing virus, HHV6 penetrates a cell, and within a few days of the invasion, the cell deteriorates to a pile of debris. Nonetheless, researchers remain cautiously optimistic that HHV6 will prove to play a significant role in chronic fatigue syndrome, although they warn against jumping to unproven conclusions. "We don't want to give patients false hopes," warns Dharam Ablashi, a herpes virologist at the National Cancer Institute. "All we can say is that HHV6 warrants further scrutiny."

Cytomegalovirus (CMV). Although the Epstein-Barr virus is the cause of classic acute mononucleosis, a cytomegalovirus infection can create very similar symptoms, including fatigue, swollen lymph glands, and fever. Like EBV, CMV is very common in the American population and initial infection is usually mild or completely asymptomatic. However, in weak or vulnerable people, CMV can wreak great damage. Babies born to mothers who become infected during pregnancy sometimes have severe congenital problems, including retardation, deafness, jaundice, or pneumonia. A CMV virus can reactivate in immunosuppressed patients, such as persons with AIDS and those who have received organ transplants, and it can be life-threatening.

Because active CMV and EBV infections look much the same, researchers speculate that if a link between the Epstein-Barr virus and chronic fatigue syndrome is proven, a similar link with cytomegalovirus probably exists.

Other Viral Suspects

A number of other viruses have been fingered as suspects in chronic fatigue syndrome. Again, none are likely to be the sole cause, but alone or in conjunction with other viruses any could trigger an infection that the body cannot control.

- Adenoviruses infect the upper respiratory tract and sometimes the stomach or intestines. Thirty-one adenoviruses are known to infect human beings; the type that causes colds, fevers, sore throats, eye and ear infections, and sometimes pneumonia may play a role in CFS.

- Enteroviruses, which enter the body through the gastrointestinal tract, have been a key focus of British research. In particular, the coxsackie B virus, known to cause blistering sore throat, intestinal infection, cough, and diarrhea, is being scrutinized.

- Retroviruses, so named because they reverse the usual sequence by which genetic information is passed along, have gained notoriety since one of its members, the human immunodeficiency virus (HIV), was identified as the cause of AIDS. New research published in 1991 showed that a high percentage of CFS patients had evidence of a retrovirus in their blood but the significance of that finding remains uncertain.

The Role of Stress and Depression

Amidst the many controversies engendered by chronic fatigue syndrome, little stirs as much heated debate as this question: What role do stress and depression play in chronic fatigue syndrome? Listen to just two opinions along the continuum: "It happens in stressful periods of already stressful lives," says Dr. Edwin Jacobson. "Patients do themselves a disservice by becoming defensive and so resistant to the idea that there is a strong psychological component to this thing."

Counters San Francisco Bay area internist Carol Jessup:

> When a woman comes in with an illness like this, it is always, always, always attributed to stress and depression, to an inability to cope with her life. It has been well-documented that women's complaints of any sort—be they headache, chest pain, abdominal pain, but particularly fatigue, are evaluated slower and less aggressively than a man who goes into the office and makes the same complaints. I never give a single

lecture on this syndrome without someone standing up and saying, "but don't you think that all these gals are just depressed?"

We can't lay this controversy to rest until CFS is better understood but it can be said with certainty that many of the high achievers who have been the most visible victims of chronic fatigue syndrome readily identify piercing stress points in their lives. It is also well known that stress plays a role in any chronic illness. "I think stress exacerbates the symptoms of this illness in the same way that it exacerbates high blood pressure, asthma, or ulcers," says Dr. Neil Singer of San Francisco. "No one thinks ulcers or asthma is a totally psychological disease. They are medical diseases that can be exacerbated by stress."

If the debate about stress ignites sparks, hinting that CFS is a physical manifestation of depression is akin to tossing a match into a can of gasoline. Dr. David Bell, who has been involved in chronic fatigue syndrome studies since illness broke out in his remote farm community of Lyndonville, New York, balks at the provocative notion. "Diagnosing someone with fever and joint pain as depressed is poor medicine," says Bell, noting that while CFS and depression share some of the symptoms—particularly fatigue, sleep disorders, headaches, and appetite changes—others differ markedly. "If depression were an unknown illness, that would be one thing, but it is not. We know a great deal about depression, it has been studied extensively." Bell suspects physicians sometimes bandy about the label of depression because they are reluctant to admit the limitations of their knowledge about CFS.

Dr. Stephen Straus of the National Institute of Allergy and Infectious Diseases is not so sure. "Everyone who deals with this syndrome professionally recognizes depression among many patients," he points out. But the significance of that observation remains unclear. According to Dr. Straus:

> One possibility is that these people are depressed because they are sick and tired of being tired and having a limited life. Or there may be chemical or metabolic mechanisms that are part of whatever is causing the syndrome that can make people depressed. If so, depression is not necessarily a reaction to their situation but an aspect of the syndrome just as fever would be.

A third alternative, adds Straus, is that many CFS patients were in fact depressed before they ever got sick and that depression does represent a risk factor for chronic fatigue syndrome.

Despite his interest in the links between depression and CFS, Dr. Straus resents any suggestion that he is skeptical about the existence of the disorder: "To say that there is a psychiatric component to this illness is not to say that it is not real," he emphasizes.

Whether or not stress and depression are ultimately shown to have a significant causative role in chronic fatigue syndrome, it is safe to say that they worsen its symptoms. An important new field of research known as psychoneuroimmunology is attempting to explain how. By pinpointing the mode of communication between the nervous and immune systems, scientists believe that psychoneuroimmunology can help them identify the biological and chemical basis for the mind-body connection. "We have to start thinking in terms of systems and their interdependency," said Dr. Robert Hallowitz, a family practitioner in suburban Washington, D.C. "They are married, your mind and your body. What happens to one system affects the other. You can't isolate the two."

The Environmental Component

With preservatives in the food we eat, pollutants in the air we breathe, and toxic wastes befouling our lands and beaches, it is no surprise if our bodies fail to process accumulated poisons without penalty. Coupled with the global consequences of the greenhouse effect and the growing hole in the ozone layer, which scientists fear may have a direct and damaging impact on the human immune system, the bill for the abuse to which we have subjected our environment appears to have come due. "I don't think we can divorce chronic fatigue syndrome from the phenomenon of what is going on in our planet," Dr. Hallowitz told a rapt audience at a major CFS medical conference in Newport, Rhode Island. "I think it is payback time, ladies and gentlemen. Our ecosystem is becoming increasingly unsupportive of our biology."

Although it is unlikely that a single chemical, preservative, or food ingredient is responsible for the spread of chronic fatigue syndrome, some combination of them could certainly be a cofactor. Tung oil and uncontrolled yeast infections have received the closest scrutiny in this regard and these are discussed in more detail below, but it is important to remember that the problem probably transcends specific toxins.

Tung Oil

The use of household products containing tung oil, which speeds drying and helps form protective, waterproof coatings, has been cited as a possible factor in CFS. An extract of the tung-oil tree, which is native to Southeast Asia, tung oil is commonly used in furniture polish, polyurethane, varnish, shellac, certain kinds of paints, and linoleum as well as in some rubbers, plastics, fiberboard, and printing inks.

To date, evidence that tung oil is in any way involved in chronic fatigue syndrome is strictly anecdotal—a number of patients trace the sudden onset of their illness to the purchase of new furniture or to undertaking a household project such as staining a piece of furniture or polyurethaning a floor. The scientific basis for the claim stems from the fact that tung oil contains phorbol esters, a chemical compound with known carcinogenic properties that speeds the replication of the Epstein-Barr virus in laboratory test tubes. Tung oil is in widespread use and clearly does not have deleterious effects on everyone but it may suppress the immune system and reactivate latent viruses in susceptible persons.

In 1988, a CFS patient brought a class action suit against a number of furniture polish manufacturers, including Proctor & Gamble, claiming that he became ill after inhaling tung oil. Unfortunately, the opportunity to lend credence to this theory—or to lay it to rest—vanished when the case was settled out of court. Similar suits, however, are still pending.

Candidiasis:
The Controversial Yeast Theory

One theory popularized in recent years is that an overgrowth of yeast in the intestines depresses the human immune system, thereby causing a range of illnesses, from acne, allergies, and rash to fatigue, depression, premenstrual syndrome, and migraine headaches. In *The Yeast Connection,* a best-selling book published in 1986, Dr. William G. Crook argues that the widespread use of antibiotics, birth control pills, cortisone, and other drugs, especially in conjunction with a sugar- and carbohydrate-rich diet, leaves us vulnerable to the ill effects of yeast toxins.

In the most recent edition of his book, Crook quoted one of his colleagues, Dr. Elmer Cranton, on the subject of CFS (which he refers to as chronic Epstein-Barr virus infection):

I feel that the chronic yeast condition weakens the immunity and causes EBV to recur and to become persistent. I am not certain which comes first, the chicken or the egg. That is, did the EBV lower immunity and cause a person to become more susceptible to yeast or vice versa? I am sure that it must occur in both directions.

At the moment, there is no hard medical evidence to back up the theory that chronic fatigue syndrome is caused by—or worsened as a result of—yeast infection. At least one internist, however, admitted that her initial skepticism about the theory had given way to a begrudging acceptance after she watched a number of her patients respond nicely to antiyeast medications and a yeast-free diet.

Genetic Predisposition:
All in the Family

Evidence suggests that there is a genetic predisposition to chronic fatigue syndrome. We know for certain that autoimmune disorders and allergies tend to run in families and the links between these conditions and chronic fatigue syndrome have already been discussed. Many physicians have particularly noted a family history of thyroid condition among CFS patients and have suggested that this common autoimmune illness may predispose an individual to the syndrome.

Janet Bohanon, co-director of the National Chronic Fatigue Syndrome Association, knows how devastating the illness can be to a family: She has been sick for twelve years and so have her two children, her brother, and her niece. "We all caught this thing at the same time," says Bohanon. "It was during my mother's funeral and everyone was crying a lot and hugging each other. Gradually all of us became severely ill. At first, I was convinced we were involved in something that was killing us all slowly."

Each family member fought a long and painful struggle to convince the medical community of the legitimacy of the illness. And all of them suffered in the process. Bohanon recalls:

At one point, my children simply refused to go to another doctor. They were tired of the implication that they were avoiding school. My son became a professional singer, performing in Las Vegas and Nashville, but he was too sick to hold many of the jobs he got. My brother had very severe reactions to drugs and needed to be hospitalized. We have all developed allergies over the years and we've gained a lot of weight because of the enforced inactivity.

Although stories similar to Janet Bohanon's have surfaced around the country, the hereditary dimensions of CFS are still not understood. As with other speculative theories on causality, a definitive statement awaits more scientific proof.

A Unifying Hypothesis

Path-breaking research is now underway to determine how so many different culprits—including viral infections, immune system irregularities, stress, environmental toxins, and genetic predisposition—might come together to cause chronic fatigue syndrome.

"My own feeling is that there is a sustained low-grade inflammatory reaction in the body that is producing these symptoms," says Atlanta physician Dr. Richard DuBois. "The real question is what is the cause of this sustained inflammatory reaction? Is there something wrong with the immune system that allows it to be perpetuated? Or is there a chronic stimulus that is triggering it? Is there more than one factor?"

Weaving together the strands of this chapter helps provide an answer to the questions raised by Dr. DuBois and lends support to his first statement. We've described the evidence of an overactive immune system among CFS patients: High rates of allergies, the similarities with autoimmune disorders, and speculation that cytokine levels are elevated all lend weight to this idea. But if some components of the immune system are overcharged, there is evidence that others appear to be weakened.

A healthy immune system has been compared to a sophisticated turbo engine. Such an engine has numerous settings to adjust fuel and air flow and other variables. Turning up one setting shuts off the engine while turning up a different setting revs it into high gear. In the same way, the highly complex immune system works most efficiently when some parts are activated and others are shut down, each at the appropriate time. An improperly activated system may free a latent virus or viruses to wreak infectious havoc; conversely, failure to halt operations may result in the overstimulation that can cause chronic infection. Once thrown off kilter, a self-perpetuating pattern of infection, overstimulation, and new infection might combine to create illness in a susceptible individual.

Where does stress fit into this model? We are developing an increasingly sophisticated understanding of its role in human physiology and its capacity to depress the immune system. Psychiatrist Dr. Leonard S. Zegans of the University of California at San Francisco explains:

> What we have is a presumption that the central nervous system and the immune system talk to each other through various chemical messengers. There are technical reasons that make it plausible that events in a person's life—in terms of stress, depression, or anxiety—might affect both the immune system and the cells that harbor a latent virus.

If immune abnormalities, a virus or viruses, and stress comprise the main ingredients of chronic fatigue syndrome, the recipe for illness may also include the effect of pollutants, a poor diet, or a genetic weakness. Together a synergistic effect is created. Explains Dr. Robert Hallowitz, "The more battles your immune system is engaged in, the less it will function and the more difficulty it will have maintaining dormancy over a latent virus."

Whatever its cause, the onset of chronic fatigue syndrome inevitably propels its victims into the maelstrom of an often confounding medical system. In the next chapter, we'll examine the long and strenuous odyssey patients take in their search for a diagnosis.

4

•

At Least There's
a Name:
The Search for a Diagnosis

The anxiety associated with significant symptoms that cannot be explained is unbelievably high. Just imagine that you have significant chest pains and no one can tell you what was wrong with you. You have nightmares, you think "oh my God, I've got something awful." What really helps these patients is to have some sense of what they have. They need a name, they need to know the ballpark they are playing in. The name isn't terribly comforting but at least it focuses them a little bit.

–Dr. Paul Cheney, Nalle Clinic,
Charlotte, North Carolina

The path from onset of illness to diagnosis with chronic fatigue syndrome is often a long and rocky one. Horror stories are rife. Patients tell of visiting twenty doctors without receiving satisfaction, of running up medical bills as high as $25,000 for specialized testing alone, and ultimately, of being diagnosed inaccurately with rare or fatal diseases.

Marc Iverson, president of the CFIDS Association in North Carolina, says that he visited more than 50 doctors, spent almost $250,000, and endured hundreds of sometimes painful diagnostic procedures in a seven-year search to understand his debilitating symptoms. One patient says that in a single week he was accused by one doctor of being a pest in need of psychiatric help and referred by another to Memorial Sloan-Kettering, the renowned cancer hospital in New York City, to be tested for malignancy.

Jessica P.'s travails are fairly typical.

My family doctor sent me to an infectious disease specialist and he referred me to an allergist. None of them knew what ailed me and for a year I trekked into the offices of every specialist you can name. Each one ran a different set of tests but they all came back normal. It was a relief to know I didn't have multiple sclerosis, lupus, or something worse, but the medical bills kept piling up and I was feeling sicker and sicker. I figured either I was going to die or I would read about myself in a medical journal.

Instead she read a newspaper article about the epidemic of illness in Nevada. Armed with a clipping that speculated about the role of Epstein-Barr virus, she returned to her family-care physician and asked to be tested for EBV antibodies, which proved abnormally high. More than a year after first becoming ill, Jessica received the diagnosis of chronic fatigue syndrome, freeing her at last to focus on obtaining appropriate treatment and the emotional support that was by then sorely needed.

How a Diagnosis Is Reached

In the absence of a reliable laboratory marker, chronic fatigue syndrome remains a subjective, sometimes speculative, diagnosis. But the release of an official definition by the Centers for Disease Control in March 1988 (see Appendix A) was an important stride toward the development of objective diagnostic criteria. Although the CDC's description is intentionally restrictive and research-oriented, it nonetheless goes a long way toward establishing exactly what chronic fatigue syndrome really is—and who has it. And by 1991, there was hope that a blood test could be developed that would confirm the immunological abnormalties that seem to point to a CFS diagnosis.

For now, though, CFS remains partly a *diagnosis of exclusion,* bestowed on a patient only after illnesses with a similar pattern of symptoms have been ruled out. According to the CDC, a lengthy list of other conditions—from autoimmune disease, cancer, and AIDS, to bacterial, fungal, or parasitic infections, psychiatric disorders, substance abuse, and neuromuscular, endocrine, cardiac, or blood disease—must first be eliminated on the basis of laboratory tests, a medical history, and a physical examination.

Doctors who are familiar with the peculiar amalgam of symptoms that accompany chronic fatigue syndrome say they are increasingly able to make a *diagnosis by inclusion* as well. "The more patients you see, the easier it gets. The key is to really get to know your patients and their symptoms and health history," said one internist. The guidelines supplied by the CDC also help in reaching an inclusive diagnosis. Under the agency's criteria, a patient must have persistent, debilitating fatigue severe enough to reduce or impair function below 50 percent of the level prior to becoming ill and it must have lasted for at least six months. In addition, a minimum number of signs and symptoms—including fever, sore throat, painful or swollen lymph nodes, generalized joint or muscle pain, exhaustion following exercise, headaches, cognitive problems, and sleep disturbances—must have developed concurrently with the fatigue or afterward.

Although the definition issued by the Centers for Disease Control has played an important role in garnering credibility for chronic fatigue syndrome, it has ironically spawned a new fear. Some physicians now express concern that CFS is being overdiagnosed "I don't know whether there is really an epidemic of chronic fatigue syndrome or not, but I am sure there is an epidemic of diagnoses," said one physician. Slapping on the CFS label carelessly is as risky and inappropriate as denying the syndrome's existence. "Either way you are doing a disservice to the patient because you are withholding the proper treatment," says San Francisco internist Neil Singer. "Right now it is too easy to say, 'it is CFS, I can't do anything about it, good-bye.'"

Before the Diagnosis

As Jessica P., whom we met at the beginning of this chapter, discovered, the months—for some patients it is years—before receiving the diagnosis of chronic fatigue syndrome are a time of anxiety and fear. One patient, who is also a registered nurse and a support group leader, observes: "For many, the most traumatic phase of the illness is still in obtaining a diagnosis. It is a financially devastating process and leaves patients feeling angry and vulnerable. We also see a tremendous erosion in self-confidence and self-image before diagnosis."

During this black period, a patient may find it hard to believe that a series of apparently unconnected symptoms are associated with the same condition. Confusion and self-doubt are the likely order of the day. Lacking validation for a peculiar set of symptoms, people often harbor secret fears about the true nature of their illness and may even question their sanity. "These are people who are very much cast adrift," says National Institutes of Health researcher Dr. Stephen Straus. "They are angry at physicians who can't find something wrong with them and can't give them a diagnosis and they are angry at themselves." Many patients waver between the poles of conviction and apprehension, convinced at one moment that their symptoms have an organic basis and wondering in the next whether they are all in the mind.

Understandably, one's imagination tends to run rather wild. Some patients become terrified that they have contracted an incurable or deadly disease. Others attach an exaggerated significance to every minor bruise or headache, interpreting each as a signal that health is spinning rapidly downward. "I remember crying, holding on to my internist's hands and begging him to save me," confessed Evelyn Eisgram, age seventy-three, an artist who has been sick for ten years.

The effort to reach diagnosis can be stressful for physicians, too. Whether because the illness might be more serious or more treatable than CFS, doctors repeatedly express fear of overlooking the true cause of a set of symptoms, thus saddling a patient with an improper diagnosis. Physicians are also conflicted over the wisdom and necessity of sending a patient to specialists—visits to neurologists, allergists, gastrointestinal experts, and even psychiatrists are costly and time-consuming, of course, but their medical expertise can be vital in pinpointing the true nature of an illness. "Diagnostic issues keep me awake at night," said one internist. "Believe me, I spend some nights looking at the ceiling and thinking, 'what if this patient really does have a brain tumor? Maybe I should get a brain scan tomorrow.' "

The Medical History

Many clinicians believe that taking a medical history of more than average detail is crucial if CFS is suspected because neither a standard physical examination or traditional laboratory tests can explain the severity of the symptoms.

"What a person has to say is extremely important in coming to diagnosis," says family practitioner Dr. Robert Hallowitz, who sets aside a full hour to speak with patients on their first visit. "All too often I hear patients complain 'no one listens, no one cares.' I try to communicate to patients that I'm interested in hearing every detail of their symptoms." At a CFS conference in Newport, Rhode Island, Hallowitz pleaded with his colleagues to obey one of the most important commandments of medicine: "Believe your patients," he urged.

If your physician is thorough, here's what you can expect from a detailed medical history:

- A thorough review of past health history, with an emphasis on childhood illnesses, experiences with surgery and hospitalization, allergies, significant life stress, and family disease.

- The opportunity to provide a detailed description of your symptoms. Dr. Hallowitz asks his patients to answer these questions about each symptom: When did it first occur? Where is it in the body? How long does it last? On a scale from 0 to 10, what is the worst that it gets? What is the least intensity? Where is it on the scale most of the time? What other symptoms are associated with it? What seems to trigger the symptom? What makes it better?

- A discussion of life-style. Exercise and sleep patterns, interpersonal relationships, and coping tools are all relevant to a patient's overall feeling of well-being. Diet should receive particular emphasis—alcohol, tobacco, and drug use, caffeine, sugar, and junk food consumption can all exacerbate the symptoms of CFS and their use should be thoroughly documented.

A medical history not only provides a vivid picture of a patient's illness but it also allows a doctor to lay the groundwork of trust that is so crucial to effective therapy. A physician who takes the time to listen conveys respect and concern that opens the door to an effective partnership. "The art of medicine is just as important as the science," said Dr. Hallowitz. "In this disorder, it may turn out that the art of medicine, the human side, is even more important than the science."

The Diagnostic Tests

After the medical history, your doctor will probably perform some laboratory tests in order to measure your overall health and to eliminate a number of other illnesses from consideration.

Certain screening tests provide a baseline from which to assess any changes in health status. A standard workup routinely includes a sedimentation rate, complete blood count, biochemistry profile, and urinalysis. A battery of more specialized tests can detect the presence of viral antibodies or measure cellular and immune system function, cognitive capacities, and thyroid and muscle function.

Other tests are added depending on symptoms and circumstance. For example, a patient with a lot of joint pain might be tested for a rheumatoid factor or an antinuclear antibody while a gay man is likely to be tested for hepatitis or AIDS. Someone around a lot of cats might be tested for toxoplasmosis and a patient who is overweight will probably be checked for an underlying thyroid condition. A test for Lyme disease has also become quite common in certain geographical regions.

Given the almost endless range of medical tests available today— some 1,500 of them by one count—it is a physician's responsibility to make appropriate choices. "Diagnostic tests have to be run selectively," says Beverly Hills physician Edwin Jacobson. "There are all sorts of tests you could run because this thing could be a hundred different diseases. But if you take time and are a halfway decent clinician, you can probably eliminate enough things with a history and a thorough examination. It isn't necessary to order everything for everybody."

As a patient and a health care consumer, you must also assume some responsibility for reaching and accepting a diagnosis. Don't urge your doctor to give you every laboratory test you hear about—lab work is often expensive and can also be inaccurate and misleading. Bear in mind that one of the hallmarks of chronic fatigue syndrome is monotonously normal lab test results. They don't indicate that there isn't anything wrong with you—only that a number of other medical problems can be ruled out.

With those caveats in mind, here is a description of some of the diagnostic tests frequently performed on patients whose symptoms resemble those of chronic fatigue syndrome.

Basic Screening Tests

Basic screening tests are relatively inexpensive, virtually risk-free, and quite common—for example, some 75 million sedimentation rate tests, 88 million urinalysis tests, and 50 million complete blood counts are performed in this country every year. Most family-care practitioners run these diagnostic tests in their offices as a matter of course.

Body Temperature. Body temperature is routinely measured, especially when an infection is suspected. Fever often indicates that the immune system is engaged in fighting a foreign invader; in the case of CFS, it is sometimes the only measurable sign of a hidden illness. You may be advised to record your body temperature at night and in the morning over a three-month period to determine whether it is fluctuating significantly.

Chemistry Profile. A battery of tests to analyze blood chemistry can be performed by a machine called the sequential multiple analyzer (SMA). Generally a chemistry profile is used to provide a broad overall picture of a patient's health rather than to diagnose a specific disease. SMA tests measure levels of cholesterol, protein, calcium, liver enzymes, uric acid, iron, electrolytes (sodium, potassium, chloride, and bicarbonate), glucose, and many other substances in the blood. Abnormalities in any one of these tests could suggest scores of potential health problems—or none at all.

Using the SMA to run automated, multiple blood chemistry tests is less costly than running selected tests individually but it is also less accurate. Even the apparent cost savings can be illusory because individuals with questionable results need to be retested. Some doctors opt instead to specify only those tests they believe to be relevant.

Complete Blood Count (CBC). The complete blood count provides information about red blood cells, white blood cells, and platelets. A general-purpose screening test, the CBC is particularly useful for detecting the presence of an infection or pinpointing the cause of anemia, but it is also used when a wide range of other disorders are suspected.

In a CBC, blood samples are analyzed automatically by a Coulter counter machine. Seven tests are performed to measure red blood cells, the most populous blood cell in the body; to count white blood cells, which are crucial for fighting infections; and to count platelets, which help ensure proper blood clotting. An eighth test, the peripheral smear analysis, requires the services of a lab technician, who examines all three types of blood cells through a microscope.

Erythrocyte Sedimentation Rate (ESR). More commonly known as the "sed rate," this is a very popular blood test used to screen for inflammation and infection. The ESR measures how rapidly red blood cells settle in specially marked test tubes. In the presence of an infection, the cells tend to cluster together and thus to fall further and more rapidly.

A nonspecific test, the sed rate has no single diagnostic utility; rather, abnormal values are taken as an indication that something is amiss. Normal sedimentation rates for most women younger than fifty are below 20 mm in one hour; healthy men average about 10 mm per hour.

Sed rates are commonly elevated in pregnant or menstruating women, but high rates may also indicate an autoimmune disorder, thyroid disease, chronic or acute infection, connective tissue diseases kidney disease, or a number of other medical conditions. Some CFS patients have elevated sed rates; however, a startling 40 percent of those measured in one study had sed rates below five, which is considered quite low.

Routine Urinalysis. There are some hundred different tests that can be performed on the urine but only a few are routinely used in general-purpose health screening. Urine is first observed by laboratory technicians for its color, clarity, odor, and foaminess. Normal urine can range in color from pale yellow to dark amber; traces of red, orange, brownish-yellow, or brownish-black suggests a range of health problems. Urine is usually clear with a characteristic odor; a sweet or fruity smell is often a sign of diabetes and a foul smell may signal infection. Very foamy urine is sometimes associated with liver problems.

Dipstick analysis—in which chemical-coated strips of plastic or paper are dipped into a urine sample—determines whether blood, glucose, protein, and other intruders are present. If so, physicians will usually look more closely for kidney or liver disease, infections, diabetes, or malnutrition. The dipstick is also used to measure the pH of urine. Normal urine is slightly acidic (average pH is between 5.0 and 6.0). Extremely acidic or highly alkaline urine can be associated with any number of disorders.

A special instrument called a urinometer measures the specific gravity of urine, which is the concentration of dissolved solids. Normal range is between 1.006 and 1.030. Lower specific gravity could signal kidney disease or sickle cell anemia; a higher concentration of solids is sometimes associated with fever, vomiting, diarrhea, and dehydration.

Finally, urine is examined under a microscope so that the presence of bacteria and parasites can be detected.

Other Laboratory Tests

Along with baseline screening, doctors have a range of other laboratory tests at their disposal. Some are used to exclude disorders that mimic CFS while others are used strictly for research purposes. Here's a look at what your doctor might be measuring when he draws your blood, injects you with thyroid hormones, encircles a magnet around you, or pricks you with electrodes.

The Epstein-Barr Virus Panel. The finding in the mid-1980s that many patients with unexplained fatigue had elevated antibody levels to the Epstein-Barr virus marked a historic breakthrough in scientific recognition of what has come to be called chronic fatigue syndrome. Although we now know that it is probably not the sole cause of CFS, the EBV antibody test continues to be used in some quarters.

"It's an unreliable test but it can be an indication that *something* is amiss," says San Francisco physician Neil Singer. "I'll do it in patients who report the symptoms because it gives more support to my suspicion that they have chronic fatigue syndrome. But if the test results are normal, it doesn't necessarily mean they don't have it."

The body produces four types of antibodies in response to four Epstein-Barr virus antigens in the blood. These antibody levels can tell us whether a person has ever been infected by EBV or was recently infected for the first time and whether the infection is latent or has been reactivated. Here is what a routine EBV serology panel measures:

- IgM antibodies to viral capsid antigen (VCA-IgM), which appear the first time a person is infected with EBV and indicate acute infection. IgM antibodies are usually undetectable within six months of primary infection, but may last up to twelve months.

- IgG antibodies to viral capsid antigen (VCA-IgG), which peak within a few weeks of an infection but remain detectable for life.

- Diffuse and restricted antibodies to early antigens (EA-D and EA-R), which appear shortly after the IgM and IgG antibodies. They can be detected in the majority of patients with acute mononucleosis and also indicate the recurrence of an EBV infection.

- Antibodies to EBV nuclear antigen (EBNA), which appear late in the course of an infection (from one to three months afterward) and theoretically persist for life.

It was the finding that chronic fatigue syndrome patients sometimes have elevated antibody levels to VCA or EA and unusually low EBNA antibodies that initially lent credence to the theory that CFS was caused by an active, recurring Epstein-Barr virus infection. However, it has since been shown that the EBV serology panels of CFS patients are not predictable and that a significant number of healthy adults have atypically high EBV antibodies. Further, elevated EBV antibody levels can be seen in patients with a number of other diseases, including AIDS, Hodgkin's disease, leukemia, rheumatoid arthritis, Burkitt's lymphoma, chronic lung disease, multiple sclerosis, and lupus. Older people and women in their third trimester of pregnancy also frequently have high levels of these antibodies. Another major problem with the EBV panel is that it is extremely hard to standardize: Lab analyses are very subjective and differ markedly from one laboratory to another and even within the same lab.

Nonetheless, in the absence of a single marker test, and despite its evident deficiencies, the EBV serology panel is likely to continue to be one weapon in the arsenal with which a physician builds a case for a CFS diagnosis.

Thyroid Function Tests. Thyroid function tests are performed in order to rule out an underlying thyroid condition and because CFS patients appear prone to the development of thyroid problems in the course of their illness.

The healthy functioning of the thyroid gland, located in the neck, is critical to normal growth and development and to proper metabolic regulation. A normal thyroid manufactures T_3 and T_4 hormones in response to thyroid-stimulating hormone (TSH), which is produced by the pituitary gland in the brain. If insufficient T_3 and T_4 hormones are produced, the thyroid is underactive (hypothyroidism) and a patient may experience weight gain, fatigue, dry skin, constipation, or the sensation of being too cold. Overproduction of thyroid hormones results in hyperthyroidism, with symptoms that include weight loss, nervousness, rapid heartbeat, diarrhea, and a feeling of being overheated. Autoimmune diseases can exist in conjunction with either of these conditions. Thyroiditis, an autoimmune disease associated with hypothyroidism, has been diagnosed in a number of chronic fatigue syndrome patients.

Levels of T_3 and T_4 hormones can be directly measured by a number of different blood tests. To test the thyroid-stimulating hormone, a physician administers intramuscular doses of TSH to a patient; if the thyroid then manufactures appropriate quantities of T_3 and T_4, the source of dysfunction is likely to be in the pituitary gland, rather than in the thyroid itself. If an autoimmune disorder is suspected, a blood test is used to measure thyroid antibody levels; abnormal antibody results have been detected in some CFS patients.

Muscle Tests. Sore and achy muscles are among the most common complaints registered by CFS patients. A number of nonspecific tests are used to gauge the health of the muscles.

• Levels of aldolase—an enzyme that helps convert sugar in the muscles to energy—are measured when damage to the muscles or other body tissue is suspected. Aldolase levels rise markedly in a range of disorders, including mononucleosis, muscular dystrophy, and hepatitis.

• Creatine phosphokinase (CPK) is an enzyme released into the bloodstream almost immediately after the heart, brain, or skeletal muscles have been damaged. The CPK blood test is most commonly administered to patients suspected of having had a heart attack but it is also used when muscular disease is suspected. Increased CPK levels are associated with muscular dystrophy and hypothyroidism.

• An electromyogram (EMG) measures the electrical activity of the muscles; it is usually accompanied by nerve conduction tests and together they pinpoint the cause of muscle weakness, tingling, or pain. The test, which can cost several hundred dollars, also helps detect stress-related muscle tension or muscle weakness that is psychosomatic in origin.

During the EMG, a needle electrode is inserted into a muscle that is then stimulated by a small current of electricity so that the response of the muscles can be recorded. For the nerve conduction tests, electrodes are taped to the skin and a similar test is performed. The patient lies at rest while the tests are administered, contracting and relaxing the muscles as instructed by the technician.

• When a muscle biopsy is performed, a small piece of tissue is removed from the body and inspected in a pathology laboratory. Recent research has turned up unusual evidence of viruses, including enteroviruses and Epstein-Barr, in biopsies taken from CFS patients with extensive muscle complaints.

Neuropsychological Testing. Because chronic fatigue syndrome patients are often plagued by problems of cognition—including concentration and memory disorders and difficulty following instruction, reasoning abstractly, using language properly, and completing tasks in logical sequence—a comprehensive battery of neuropsychological tests are sometimes recommended. Administered over several sessions and designed to assess sophisticated brain functions, proper neuropsychological testing can pinpoint damage to the cerebral cortex, the outer portion of the brain that is most sensitive to viral attack.

Not all CFS patients experience cognitive problems and this battery of tests is not a mandatory part of a patient's evaluation. However, when cognitive dysfunction is present, the tests enable physicians to distinguish between neurotic or malingering patients and those with organic damage. Neuropsychological test results also serve as powerful evidence in support of Social Security disability claims, discussed elsewhere in this book. A magnetic resonance imaging (MRI) scan is usually indicated if the tests are significantly abnormal.

Magnetic Resonance Imaging (MRI). The magnetic resonance imaging scanner is a revolutionary new diagnostic tool that produces more detailed images of the body's internal organs than is possible with an X-ray or any other imaging technique. To obtain an MRI scan, the patient is placed inside a machine that contains a large magnet. A magnetic pulse is then sent out that causes the nuclei of certain hydrogen atoms in the body to point in the same direction; when the pulse stops, the atoms return to their normal position while emitting an electrical echo. That echo is then converted into a detailed image of the area.

MRI tests are costly—running in the neighborhood of $1,000 per test—but they are usually covered by good health insurance policies. Under certain circumstances, they are more informative than either X-rays or computerized axial tomography (CAT) scans, and are particularly appropriate for patients with allergies, who may react to the injectable dye used in a CAT scan. Painless and virtually risk-free, MRIs are being used widely in medicine today to diagnose everything from torn ligaments to multiple sclerosis and brain tumors.

Their use in the diagnosis of chronic fatigue syndrome is highly controversial, however. A number of physicians who regularly use MRIs to scan the brain tissue of CFS patients report finding lesions, marked by unusual bright spots, that may indicate inflammation or some form of organic brain damage. Researchers disagree as to whether there is a link between these findings and the cognitive problems so common among CFS patients. "The lesions we see with the MRI may not themselves be causing a problem, but they represent something that is," says Dr. Paul Cheney, one of the clinicians who first broke the story of the Incline Village, Nevada, epidemic. Anaheim Hills physician Jay Goldstein agrees: "We don't really know what the bright objects mean. They are not diagnostic of the disease but when you see really large ones in a young person that is highly suspicious."

Other physicians are not so sure. Similar findings have been reported in healthy people and there is speculation that the bright spots are part of a natural aging process or an indication of a past head injury that has no bearing on present illness. The significance of the MRI scans therefore remains uncertain.

Excluding Other Autoimmune Diseases.

As we discussed earlier, a link is suspected between chronic fatigue syndrome and autoimmune disorders. Because CFS shares symptomatic similarities with lupus, rheumatoid arthritis, multiple sclerosis, and thyroiditis, tests to rule out these autoimmune diseases are quite common. Significantly, a small number of CFS patients show somewhat abnormal results on one or more of the following tests but manifest no other sign of these diseases.

- Antinuclear antibody testing (ANA) is generally done when lupus is suspected or when a number of unexplained symptoms are present, including arthritic pain, skin rash, or chest pain. An easy-to-perform blood test, ANA values may be higher than normal in the presence of several autoimmune diseases or when there is a viral infection. Some healthy individuals also have unusually high ANAs.

- Rheumatoid factor is the standard blood test for rheumatoid arthritis, which causes inflamed, painful, and stiff joints. However, higher than normal lab results may also signal lupus, polio, tuberculosis, mononucleosis, syphilis, or liver, lung, or heart conditions. A number of other symptoms must be present to confirm a rheumatoid arthritis diagnosis.

- Thyroiditis, or inflammation of the thyroid, can be tested with thyroid antibody blood tests, which are discussed above.

- While there is no single laboratory test for multiple sclerosis, the MRI's capacity to identify and record brain lesions has made the diagnosis of MS much easier. Important information is also collected with the use of an electroencephalograph (EEG), which measures the brain's electrical response to visual, auditory, and pain stimulation. A spinal tap, once a routine part of an MS diagnosis, is no longer standard procedure.

Specialized Immune System Tests. As scientific understanding of the immune system grows, it has become increasingly easier to measure specific components of immunological functioning, most commonly using easy-to-obtain blood samples. These highly specialized—and often quite costly—lab tests are not generally recommended as a matter of course for CFS patients but they are sometimes used for research purposes or to rule out other disorders:

- Lymphocyte phenotyping involves detecting and differentiating the white blood cells of the immune system. These tests have allowed researchers to detect subtle abnormalities in the helper/suppressor T-cell ratio and in natural killer cells.

- Kappa/lambda clonal excess analysis detects the proliferation of specially marked B lymphocytes, which can signal a lymphoproliferative disorder.

- Lymphokine tests can detect the presence of elevated levels of the interferon and interleukin proteins. Normally present while the body is fighting a viral infection, prolonged elevation can indicate an overactive immune system.

- Laboratory tests also measure levels of circulating immune complexes, immunoglobulin molecules and cellular-mediated immunity. In some individuals ultimately diagnosed with CFS, immune complex levels are somewhat elevated, although still below those typically associated with immune complex diseases. Suppressed immunoglobulin secretion has also been shown to be consistent with a diagnosis of chronic fatigue syndrome. The Multitest CMI device, in which the skin is pricked with antigens so that its response can be observed, is used to measure cell-mediated immunity. Some CFS patients are *hypoergic* (reduced CMI) or *anergic* (absent CMI).

After the Diagnosis

Once the results of all appropriate lab tests are analyzed, then added to the findings from the physical exam and the medical history, a physician familiar with the multiple manifestations of chronic fatigue syndrome will feel reasonably confident about pronouncing a diagnosis. What happens next?

As a patient you will most likely feel enormously relieved simply to have a name assigned to your disquieting collection of symptoms. Knowing that the vague, sometimes bizarre, symptoms have their origins in a very real illness is the critical first step toward obtaining proper care. While the chronic fatigue syndrome diagnosis is hardly a friendly one, the assurance that your condition is unlikely to deteriorate or prove fatal has healing properties of its own.

Still a wave of depression washes over many CFS patients as they begin to grasp the realities of grappling with a mystifying and chronic illness. Anger at the pace of your recovery and at the limitations imposed on your once full and happy life is only natural. Depending on your support systems, you may also suffer isolation because family, friends, and co-workers cannot fully grasp the depth of your illness and guilt since you cannot meet their expectations.

Learning to accept a diagnosis as uncertain as chronic fatigue syndrome does not come quickly or easily. Indeed it is said that one mourns the loss of one's good health in much the same way that one mourns the loss of a loved one, a process that is discussed in detail later in this book. Most patients agree, however, that learning to accept the reality of a chronic illness is crucial to regaining a sense of control over their lives.

Once you have been diagnosed, it is important to remain in close touch with a primary-care physician who understands CFS and knows that every ache and pain you describe cannot necessarily be attributed to the primary disorder. Even if the diagnosis of CFS is an accurate one, there is no guarantee that unrelated problems won't present themselves at a future date. To assume that each one is inevitably linked to CFS is risky and could mean you won't get the care you need. That's exactly what happened to Shawn R. Certain that his worsening fatigue and dizziness were just another manifestation of CFS, he neglected to call his internist until the symptoms simply became overpowering. After a quick examination, he was admitted to the hospital, where further tests revealed a life-threatening internal hemorrhage entirely unrelated to chronic fatigue syndrome.

Along with monitoring your health, primary-care physicians have a number of treatment alternatives at their disposal. While there is no cure for CFS, specific symptoms can be relieved if your doctors know what's bothering you most and which medications seem to help. Chronic fatigue syndrome is neither static nor predictable, and as the nature and severity of symptoms shift, it may be appropriate for you to experiment with new forms of treatment. In the next chapter, we'll look at the range of options available and discuss the help you can reasonably expect from your physician or health care provider.

5

■

Until the Cure Comes:
Treatment That Makes
a Difference

We have people in droves who cannot wait until we have the answers to all our questions before we begin to intervene. It is your moral duty to apply all the knowledge that you have gained in service to your patients, observing first the dictum, do no harm.

–Dr. Robert Hallowitz, family medicine practitioner,
Gaithersburg, Maryland, addressing a
medical conference

There is no remedy for the condition but simply knowing there is an organic explanation for their distressing symptoms, that it is not all in their minds, brings significant relief to most patients.

–Jane Brody, health writer,
New York Times

Coming to grips with the limitations of medical science is one of the toughest tasks any chronically ill patient must face. Most of us have been raised to believe in the powers of technology and the breadth of our physician's knowledge. To discover that there are certain ailments neither one can cure is disheartening and disillusioning. Yet the hard-to-handle fact remains that there is no known cure for chronic fatigue syndrome as of yet.

Still there is much that patients can do to improve the state of their health as they work closely with informed and compassionate physicians. Treatment is highly individualized with no single regimen appropriate for everyone. Some patients have shown marked improvement by adjusting the tempo of their lives, taking appropriate prescription and over-the-counter medications to relieve symptoms, and experimenting, under close medical supervision, with a range of other therapies. Principles of sound nutrition, the use of vitamins, minerals, and holistic health remedies, intensive rest, and practical techniques to ease the daily pressures of life have also boosted energy levels and improved the functional capacity of many CFS patients.

Unfortunately finding effective treatment for chronic fatigue syndrome remains largely a trial-and-error process. And so it will be until scientists and medical researchers can agree on just what triggers CFS. The problem is that if we don't know whether illness is caused by a virus, the effectiveness of antiviral medications is strictly speculative; similarly, without understanding the pathway that connects allergic reactions to the syndrome, we can't be sure how useful allergy medications really are.

The Search for Appropriate
Health Care

The frankly bizarre and seemingly unrelated constellation of symptoms that often characterize CFS still draw skepticism from the medical community, especially from physicians who have not been confronted by them before. And the fact that the scientific community has only begun to understand the illness has further heightened the reluctance to deal with it. "Physicians are enormously frustrated by any condition they can't help. It's hard just to treat symptoms and remain in the dark about a cause," acknowledges one Atlanta physician.

There's another reason that chronic fatigue syndrome patients have sometimes received short shrift—and it does not cast a flattering light on the medical profession. According to Dr. Edwin Jacobson of Beverly Hills, CFS patients require a lot of time and attention but doctors can't make a lot of money from them. This internist explains:

> These are not the kind of patients physicians see if they want to build a large practice, get patients in and out the door in fifteen minutes. There is no easy procedure you can do—you can't cure this with an operation or a shot. Unless they have a personal interest in patients with problems like this, most doctors will give poor service to them.

Fortunately the growing numbers of journal articles, the availability of private and public research dollars, and the interest that has been expressed in CFS by Congress have begun to enhance the credibility and prestige of being involved with chronic fatigue syndrome. This interest, in turn, is piquing physician interest, making it much easier to find someone who is informed, sympathetic, and fascinated by the illness. Increasingly, doctors have realized that as frustrating as CFS can be to treat, it also offers tremendous challenge and opportunity to the intellectually curious. "This is a training ground for the art of medicine," notes Dr. James Jones, the pioneering CFS investigator connected with the National Jewish Center for Immunology and Respiratory Medicine in Denver, Colorado.

Selecting a Primary-Care Physician

Because chronic fatigue syndrome has potential implications for all of the body's major systems, internists or family-care practitioners generally have the broad-based background most appropriate for providing treatment. Infectious disease specialists, subspecialists of internal medicine, and clinical immunologists are also seeing significant—and growing—numbers of patients.

There's no point in expending precious energy—to say nothing of precious dollars—in a mad dash from one physician to another in desperate hope of finding a miracle drug to vanquish your health woes. Instead it is better to select a primary-care physician with whom you feel some rapport and stay in regular touch so that he or she is alert to any changes in your condition. "We need an old-fashioned country doctor who will really listen to our symptoms," said one support group leader in Dallas, Texas. If it becomes appropriate to consult specialists for particular symptoms, ask your primary-care physician for referrals. And be sure to report back on what the specialists suggest, particularly if new medications are prescribed for you.

Most local support groups maintain referral lists of local doctors. In New York, for example, the list includes a fee schedule, information about insurance, and whether the doctor is willing to make house calls. The CFIDS Association in North Carolina maintains a nationwide "physician's honor roll," based on patient recommendations, which is a valuable aid in finding sympathetic medical care. The National CFS Association in Kansas City, Missouri, urges patients whose internists are unschooled in the enigma of chronic fatigue syndrome to share current medical literature with them. "If you can educate your family doctor, that is to the benefit of hundreds that come behind you," says Janet Bohanon, vice-president of the association.

A word of caution about selecting appropriate health care is sadly in order. "There are a lot of opportunists in this field," warns Dr. Nathaniel Brown, a pediatric infectious disease specialist at North Shore University Hospital in the New York City suburb of Manhasset, Long Island. "It is exactly in an area like chronic fatigue syndrome, where you have vague complaints but people are unlikely to die, that charlatans arise. The treatment they offer is usually harmless, ineffective, and costly."

What You Can Expect from Your Physician

No matter what physicians can—and cannot—offer you in the way of help, they should be expected to treat you with respect, compassion, and the benefit of the latest medical knowledge. Unfortunately it cannot yet be said that all physicians do so. "Some of our patients have been mocked for having a 'yuppie disease' and have left the doctor's office in tears," says Janet Bohanon.

Here is what you can reasonably expect from a primary-care physician:

- A willingness to listen. Doctors certainly don't have all the answers to your complaints but they've got to take the time to hear about them and to respond with suggestions, observations, and when appropriate, with new treatments.

- Familiarity with the latest research in the field. New information is rapidly emerging about the treatment of chronic fatigue syndrome and it is important that your physician remain current as the findings are published.

- A conviction that chronic fatigue syndrome has an organic basis and that symptoms may respond to medical treatment. Some doctors, including ones who regularly treat CFS patients, still believe that the elimination of stress is the sole obstacle to recovery. Seek out a physician who understands that regardless of cause, medical intervention may be necessary once CFS gains a toehold in your body.

• The time to see you regularly. Chronic fatigue syndrome is not a static condition; as symptoms wax and wane in severity, a thorough physician will want to change your medications and emphasize different treatments for your most debilitating symptoms. Any doctor who closes the book on your case once a CFS diagnosis has been made is not serving you properly.

• An open mind and a concern for the fact that other diseases can exist concurrently with CFS. Unfortunately, having CFS provides no assurance that you won't sicken with another, entirely unrelated, illness. It is easy for your physician to assume that any complaint is linked to chronic fatigue syndrome but obviously that's not always the case. Your doctor should check you out thoroughly whenever your condition changes significantly.

• Knowledge of the multidisciplinary services you may need. Along with providing you with health care, your physician should be able and willing to make appropriate referrals for psychological counseling, physical therapy, stress reduction, nutrition counseling, and social welfare programs, such as Social Security disability.

The best health care results from a cooperative patient–physician partnership. As a patient, you've got some responsibilities, too. Prior to every visit with your physician, you should make some notes that will help you describe your illness in an organized and coherent fashion. A diary prepared expressly for CFS patients by Dr. Arnold Goldberg in Ontario, Canada (see Appendix B) allows you to record your personal health and allergy history, medication and treatment experiences, and relapses and their possible causes. A monthly self-assessment sheet is also provided.

Be prepared with questions so that you don't leave the doctor's office feeling more confused than when you first arrived. And don't bristle if inquiries are made about your emotional state or if questions about stress and depression are raised: These are perfectly legitimate avenues of inquiry designed to develop an overall picture of your health. Rely on your own instincts, though. If you sense that your doctor really doesn't accept the legitimacy of chronic fatigue syndrome, look elsewhere for health care.

From the Medicine Cabinet

In the absence of a clear-cut treatment regimen for chronic fatigue syndrome, physicians are doing a great deal of experimenting on their own. Scores of medications—some to relieve specific symptoms, others theorized to bolster the immune system—are under scrutiny. Unfortunately the very fact that so many different drugs are rumored to be helpful is evidence that a definitive cure remains elusive. And very few treatments being used have been subjected to the rigorous standards of scientific experimentation: double-blind studies in which one patient population receives a test medication while another receives a placebo, and where neither scientist nor patient know who has received which one. Until that sort of replicable research is done, the effectiveness of most CFS treatment remains highly speculative.

"I'm trying everything," said one internist in exasperation, adding that frontline doctors, who treat dozens or even hundreds of CFS patients, are in dire need of more uniform treatment guidelines. Another physician in private practice likened his treatment regimen to a Chinese menu:

> Column A are the drugs that bring symptomatic relief, easing inflammation, low-grade aches and pains, and sleep disorders. Column B are heavier-duty drugs, such as the antiviral medications. Column C are more unorthodox remedies thought to enhance the immune system's ability to fight off illness. I recommend treatments in each of these categories on a trial and error basis.

Dr. Jay Goldstein, who has a specialized clinic for CFS patients in Beverly Hills, California, has developed a "ladder of treatment" that begins with the least costly, least risky treatments and ascends toward more potent medications if the others prove ineffective or inadequate. A specialist in patients who are difficult to diagnose and hard to treat, Goldstein tells people with chronic fatigue syndrome, "There is a good chance I can make you feel considerably better so you will be able to function. But if you were used to working real long hours or doing superhuman feats, it is not likely that I will be able to improve you to that point."

Along with a range of over-the-counter and prescription medications, which are described in detail below, most doctors provide common sense, Marcus Welby-style advice: Rest when necessary; eat a balanced diet; exercise, if possible, but at a level that does not intensify fatigue; learn to pace yourself to reduce stress; and make the life-style adjustments necessary to cope with your greatly lessened energy level. Reassurance is an important part of long-range treatment. In it worst phases, CFS symptoms are debilitating and bizarre and patients need regular reminders that the illness generally does not progress to something more serious and that in time they will begin to feel better.

As we discuss the medications being used to treat chronic fatigue syndrome patients, remember:

- *The treatments described here are not endorsements; we don't recommend specific therapeutic modalities.* The information is provided only to help you make informed decisions about your health care. It is never appropriate to self-medicate. All treatments, even over-the-counter medicines, should be selected in consultation with your doctor.

- Many CFS patients are unable to tolerate the full recommended dose of medication because of allergic reactions from chemical sensitivities. Your physician may initially prescribe a one-quarter dose, then increase it gradually to find the optimal level that is both effective and tolerable.

- Sensitivities to the dyes used to coat tablet medications are quite common and many doctors prefer liquid medication or noncoated capsules, when they are available.

- As a health care consumer, you have the right to be fully informed about potential drug side effects, dangerous interactions, and the possibility that taking one medication increases or decreases the effects of others. Some potential hazards are mentioned here but there may be others. Unfortunately, doctors are often shockingly ignorant about pharmacology. To be safe, talk with your pharmacist or consult the *Physicians' Desk Reference (PDR)* (Medical Economics) or *U.S. Pharmacopeia Drug Information* (U.S. Pharmacopeial Convention), the two bibles of medication. If the medication is too new to be listed, you can ask your health care provider for the information that is supplied by the manufacturer.

- Keep a log of the medications you are taking, especially if you see more than one doctor or have memory problems. Along with helping you remember what medicines to take, and when, the log may help pinpoint the cause of new or changed symptoms. Carry this record with you whenever you see a physician and leave a copy with your pharmacist.

• Given the high percentage of adverse drug reactions among CFS patients, stay alert to even mild side effects and tell your doctor about them immediately. You may also want to ask for samples or a small supply of a new medicine so that you don't waste money on a drug you can't tolerate.

Painkillers and Anti-Inflammatory Medication

Treating pain is a tricky business because it is so subjective: Doctors have no way of measuring it or comparing the extent of your pain with that of another patient. For this reason, they are likely to experiment with pain relievers, trying first one, then another medication, alone or in low-dose combinations, until they find the most effective treatment possible. Although pain medication relieves only the symptoms, not the cause, of chronic pain, it can play a vital role in helping you live a more normal life.

For sore throat, achy joints and muscles, mild inflammations, and headache and body tenderness, aspirin remains one of the safest, most effective, over-the-counter medications available. Check the ingredients list on the aspirin you buy and avoid brands with added caffeine if they don't agree with you. If aspirin irritates your stomach you may wish to try a buffered product. Although it does not reduce inflammation, acetaminophen (Tylenol is the best-known brand name) is as effective as aspirin for the relief of pain. CFS patients have also found ibuprofen (Advil and Motrin are common brand names) to be effective, particularly for severe joint pain. Ibuprofen should not be taken in conjunction with aspirin or acetaminophen.

A wide range of other pain relievers and anti-inflammatory medications are available by prescription. Naproxen, sold under the brand names Naprosyn and Anaprox, is a commonly used analgesic. Mild narcotics such as codeine or propoxyphene (Darvon is the best-known brand name), and combination drugs such as Fiorinal (which contains aspirin, caffeine, codeine, and the sedative butalbital), have also proved effective. Some physicians prescribe steroids to reduce severe joint inflammation but these are potent medications with highly toxic side effects and should never be used casually or for pain only.

Antidepressants

Uncomfortable with any hint that CFS has its roots in psychological depression, many patients are initially reluctant to take antidepressant medication. At the low doses prescribed for the treatment of the syndrome, however, antidepressants work to restore a proper chemical balance in the brain, rather than to cure depression linked to emotional problems. They are also commonly used in the treatment of balance disorders. "Antidepressants work not because they are 'happy pill,' because they are not, and not because they in some way change the person, which they don't," said Dr. Edwin Jacobson. "What antidepressants do for CFS patients is change the balance of the neurotransmitters (the chemical messengers of the nerve cells) in their head."

Antidepressants in two major families—the tricyclic group and the monoamine oxidase (MAO) inhibitors—are coming under the closest scrutiny in the treatment of chronic fatigue syndrome, although others are in use as well. At conventional doses, many of these drugs can cause a number of unpleasant side effects including weight gain, dry mouth, blurred vision, sedation, and constipation, but at the dosages normally recommended for CFS patients, these problems are less likely to occur.

Tricyclic Antidepressants. The development of a class of antidepressants known as the tricyclics represented a major breakthrough in the treatment of classic depression in the 1960s and 1970s. Two tricyclics in particular—Sinequan (generic name, doxepin) and Elavil (generic name, amitriptyline)—are being highlighted for use in CFS.

Results with both Sinequan and Elavil have been promising with patients reporting a boost in their energy levels and improved sleep patterns. Sinequan has powerful antihistamine and anti-inflammatory effects as well, which make it effective as a pain reliever and particularly appropriate for patients with allergies. According to Dr. James Jones of the National Jewish Center for Immunology and Respiratory Medicine in Denver, Sinequan relieves symptomatic discomfort for 70 percent of CFS patients.

Typically the antidepressant dose given to chronic fatigue syndrome patients is a fraction of that used to treat classic depression. For example, depressed patients usually start with 50 mg/day of Sinequan and build to 150–200 mg/day. CFS patients, by contrast, start with only 10 mg/day to a maximum of 50–75 mg/day. Although physicians do not understand why, some CFS patients can tolerate only doses of 5 mg/day or less of the drug yet are helped by these minute quantities. If improvement is not evident within five to seven weeks, antidepressant therapy is discontinued.

Anyone who has been using the MAO inhibitor drugs, described below, needs to wait at least two weeks before trying a tricyclic antidepressant.

Monoamine oxidase (MAO) inhibitors. Monoamine oxidase inhibitors, which inhibit the monoamine oxidase enzyme in the nervous system, are traditionally used to combat depression that manifests itself in anxiety and psychosomatic symptoms. The most common MAOs are Nardil (generic name, phenelzine sulfate) and Parnate (generic name, tranylcypromine sulfate).

Nardil was successfully used in one small trial of CFS patients: Seventeen out of twenty-one people responded to the medication with at least some significant improvement in their energy levels. However, there are a number of potentially dangerous food and drug interactions with Nardil and your physician should warn you about these. In particular, the drug cannot be used in conjunction with antihistamines, anticonvulsants, muscle relaxants, and certain pain medications and tranquilizers. Eating foods with a high tyramine content, including cheese, certain meat products, and overripe fruits, can be dangerous: Be sure your doctor gives you a list of prohibited foods and beverages.

Antiviral Medications

Despite tremendous medical advances, scientists continue to be stymied by viruses. Unlike bacteria-linked disease, which can often be treated with antibiotics, there is no cure for an extraordinarily long list of viral illnesses, from AIDS to influenza. The crux of the treatment problem is that viruses are so intimately involved with the human cell that most medication has toxic effects. Indeed it is largely because effective treatment has been difficult to find for such viral diseases as polio, smallpox, measles, and hepatitis that medical research has focused on prevention via the development of vaccinations.

The fact that a specific virus has not been identified as the certain cause of chronic fatigue syndrome further complicates the use of antiviral medications. Nonetheless, several important drugs are under evaluation.

Zovirax. Better known by the generic name of acyclovir, the drug was heralded as a major breakthrough in efforts to treat genital herpes and became widely available in the early 1980s. It has also proven to be effective in inhibiting the replication of other viruses in the herpes class. When the Epstein-Barr virus was the chief viral suspect in chronic fatigue syndrome, many physicians began to treat their patients with aggressive doses of acyclovir.

Although anecdotal reports of acyclovir use by CFS patients were promising, results of 1987 and 1988 studies by Dr. Stephen E. Straus, the National Institutes of Health virologist, were disappointing. In a double-blind experiment, nineteen women and eight men received either high doses of acyclovir (administered intravenously for seven days, then orally for a month) or a placebo. Patients receiving acyclovir then switched to a placebo; those receiving the placebo were given acyclovir. When results were ultimately analyzed, no meaningful difference was found between the effectiveness of acyclovir and the placebo.

Some physicians argue, however, that the results of the Straus study are not conclusive for *all* CFS patients. Acyclovir is still commonly prescribed in large does (up to 800 mg daily), especially when the illness has been identified in its early stages. Intravenous acyclovir is expensive and sometimes causes light-headedness, headaches, and in rare cases adverse renal or hematological (blood-related) effects. In most clinical practices, the capsule form of acyclovir is recommended, but unpleasant side effects include diarrhea, dizziness, headaches, and joint pain.

Given the mixed reports on the effectiveness of acyclovir, further studies are clearly necessary. Meanwhile, it is appropriate to discuss its use with your physician.

Symmetrel. Symmetrel (generic name, amantadine) is an antiviral drug that is used against the A strain of influenza and also in the treatment of Parkinson's disease. Recently it has been prescribed for chronic fatigue syndrome in the hopes that it will counteract low-grade inflammation; its effectiveness has not yet been proven. Side effects of Symmetrel can include light-headedness, insomnia, and concentration problems, although these have not been widely reported among CFS patients.

Gamma Globulin Therapy

Gamma globulin, also called immunoglobulin, contains a mixture of antibodies and is being used by some physicians to bolster the immune system of CFS patients and to provide temporary symptomatic relief. Made from human blood, gamma globulin treatment has three interrelated benefits: First, it contains antibodies that kill viruses in the bloodstream before they can penetrate a cell; second, it alerts the body's T cells to the presence of infected B cells, so they can be killed; and third, it provides a specific antibody that is thought to be missing in CFS patients.

Some physicians opt for less costly intramuscular (IM) gamma globulin injections; others believe intravenous (IV) injections are more effective. Typically, a patient receives an intramuscular injection once a week for four weeks and then returns for additional shots on an as-needed basis, anywhere from two weeks to three months apart. Before gamma globulin injections begin, patients must be tested to reduce the likelihood of an allergic reaction.

Unfortunately gamma globulin is not a cure for CFS: Not every patient who tries gamma globulin shows any sign of improvement, and even among those who do, symptoms return in full force as soon as the injections are stopped. A study of the effectiveness of gamma globulin therapy in conjunction with acyclovir is being conducted at the National Cancer Institute.

Ulcer Medications

Tagamet (generic name, cimetidine) and Zantac (generic name, ranitidine) are H-2 receptor blockers traditionally prescribed in the treatment of peptic ulcers. H-2 blockers inhibit the action of histamine and thus the secretion of stomach acid, thereby allowing ulcers to heal. The hope for CFS patients is that H-2 blockers will also inhibit the overproduction of lymphokines, the naturally occurring chemicals of the immune system that may cause some of the flu-like symptoms of illness.

Results to date have been promising: H-2 receptor blockers have temporarily lessened the fatigue and reduced the intensity of a number of symptoms associated with CFS in a number of patients, although these return when the medication is halted. Cimetidine and ranitidine have also been used effectively for patients who are bothered by gastritis, an inflammation in the stomach membrane, and have eased the problems of vomiting or nausea sometimes associated with CFS.

Tagamet and Zantac are considered relatively safe drugs when taken alone but in conjunction with other medications they can have serious side effects. Both drugs should be administered with caution if you are also taking anticoagulants, anticonvulsants, or asthma medication; ask your doctor about the possibility of dangerous interactions. Tagamet should not be taken in combination with antidepressant medications, such as Sinequan. A sudden withdrawal from Zantac can cause a severe reaction so consult with your doctor about ways to cut back gradually.

Treatment for Sleep Disorders

Providing medications or other remedies that help you obtain a good night's sleep works wonders for an individual's sense of well-being and is sometimes the most valuable service a physician can perform. The low doses of antidepressants we've already described improve sleep patterns but other treatments are available as well

Over-the-Counter Medications. The active ingredient of most over-the-counter sleep medications is antihistamine, traditionally used in the relief of cold and allergy symptoms. Cope, Sominex, Sleep-Eze, Compoz, Nytol, and scores of other brand-name sleep products are likely to contain one or more of these antihistamines: doxylamine, diphenhydramine, or pyrilamine. Be sure to discuss the use of over-the-counter sleep medications with your doctor because of possible hazardous interactions with prescription drugs.

Prescription Drugs. Benzodiazepines, a class of minor tranquilizers of which Valium is the best known, are the drug of choice for short-term insomnia. Although they are much preferred to the more potent barbiturates, benzodiazepines are addictive. Halcion (generic name, triazolam) and Xanax (generic name, alprazolam) are commonly prescribed for CFS patients. More recently, a number of patients have reported satisfactory results with Klonopin (generic name, Clonazepan). The chief advantage of benzodiazepines is that they are short-acting so that patients are generally alert by morning; other hypnotic agents, by contrast, can leave you feeling groggy all day. Patients who are taking Tagamet (an ulcer medication described above) or over-the-counter antihistamines are advised against Halcion; the interactions can cause excessive sedation.

Another effective medication for CFS patients is Buspar (generic name, buspirone), a mild tranquilizer. Although not developed specifically as a sleeping pill, its capacity to relieve anxiety and nervous tension enables some individuals to sleep through the night. Buspar has relatively little potential for addiction but it usually takes a week or so to exert its calming effect.

Drug-Free Sleep. Unfortunately sleep medication does not treat underlying problems, and when used over a long period of time, it can actually cause insomnia rather than cure it. For this reason, volumes have been written about combating chronic insomnia without medication. Relaxation techniques, biofeedback, and self-hypnosis can all be helpful. In addition, it is wise to cut back on caffeine consumption and to avoid large meals shortly before bedtime. Regular exercise, if possible, or at least a regular dose of fresh air, is helpful, and unwinding just before going to bed—by listening to music, watching television, or reading—can slow down body function. If you lie awake tossing and turning for more than twenty minutes, try getting out of bed and sitting or reading quietly in another room before attempting to return to sleep.

More good advice about improving sleep is offered by Drs. Charles Lapp and Paul Cheney, who advise patients to follow a fixed schedule of retiring and arising and to adjust their daily schedules to accommodate their natural body rhythms. Curiously, they have found that many of their patients prefer going to bed late and then sleeping late as well.

Treatment for Vestibular Disorders

Since the mid-1980s, great strides have been made in understanding the balance problems that often plague CFS patients. Computer-age testing equipment—such as the platform and rotation chair, which was originally conceived for NASA space research programs—is now used to pinpoint vestibular disorders. Physical therapy and special educational programs to literally retrain the brain have been developed and offer new hope to previously untreatable patients.

However, unless specific neurological damage is identified, balance disorders are mostly treated symptomatically. Sedatives and antihistamines—ask for a brand that will not intensify fatigue—can reduce episodes of vertigo and panic attacks. Antinausea medications or the scopolamine patch, which is placed on the skin behind the ear to stave off motion sickness, are sometimes effective.

An imbalance in body fluid levels can contribute to vestibular problems, which helps explain why patients scmetimes crave liquids. Dietary modifications are advisable—in particular, lowering levels of salt and sugar in the diet and drinking sufficient fluids to replace those lost during exercise or hot weather can ease difficulties with balance.

Coping with Allergies

IgE-Mediated Allergies. Although the precise link between CFS and allergies is poorly understood, allergy relief can immeasurably improve the way you feel. If the source of allergies can be pinpointed, avoiding the offending allergens is the preferred mode of treatment. A wide range of antihistamine products and other mild medications provide effective symptomatic relief. Immunotherapy, in the form of desensitization shots, is used for severe allergies, especially those that could be life-threatening.

Environmental Toxins. The operating principle of clinical ecology is that the accumulated toxins contained in many common household items, food products, cosmetics, and even clothing materials can cause or exacerbate illness. As with conventional IgE-meciated allergies, avoidance is the preferred mode of treatment. Purging a home of suspected toxins can entail changing the bedding and the carpeting, reducing the use of certain personal and household cleaning products, avoiding plastics, and even changing the furnishings. Life-style changes, notably stress reduction, experimental therapies to boost the immune system, and dietary restrictions are also part of a custom-tailored clinical ecology regimen.

Food Sensitivities. Food sensitivities are a major subcategory of environmental allergies. When such sensitivities are suspected, recommended dietary changes include avoiding preservatives, minimizing consumption of processed foods, and drinking bottled rather than tap water. Particular food preparation and storage techniques and the use of certain types of pots and pans are also recommended by those who accept the controversial correlation between food sensitivity and illness. For example, meat fat should be cut away because pesticides tend to accumulate there and food should be stored in paper or foil rather than in polyurethane or plastic. Sources for further information on food sensitivities and how to treat them are included in Appendix C.

The theory that certain foods, as well as medication, can cause an overgrowth of yeast within the body has been popularized by Dr. William G. Crook in *The Yeast Connection* (Professional Books). When candidiasis is suspected, CFS patients are urged to restrict yeast consumption by limiting sugar and refined carbohydrates and avoiding vinegars and fermented products including alcohol, fruit juices, and cheese. Antibiotics, birth control pills, B-complex vitamins, and selenium, a trace element contained in many foods, should also be avoided if possible. A number of patients are taking oral mystatin to combat candidiasis.

Other Treatments

Other conventional pharmaceutical therapies being used to treat chronic fatigue syndrome patients include:

- B_{12} injections: B_{12} vitamins are essential to the maintenance of healthy nerve tissues and to cellular replication. Although serious vitamin B_{12} deficiencies are rare, some physicians report success using intramuscular injections of B_{12} to bolster overall health and heighten well-being.

- Thyroid hormones: Natural forms of thyroid hormones, usually derived from the glands of animals, are administered in capsule or tablet form to CFS patients who exhibit thyroid deficiencies. Thyroid medication has also been used to treat nonspecific fatigue, but the appropriateness of this practice is highly questionable. If your doctor finds no indication of hypothyroidism, ask careful questions about why you are being given the hormone. Common brand names for thyroid hormones include Levothroid, Synthroid, Cytomel, Euthroid, Thyrolar, and Proloid.

- Doxycycline: An antibiotic of the tetracycline class, doxycycline has been used successfully to suppress CFS symptoms. The prescription drug prevents the growth and multiplication of susceptible bacteria and curiously was initially prescribed when a bacterial cause for CFS was suspected. Researchers now hypothesize that doxycycline also suppresses the synthesis of interleukin-2, a natural immune system substance that may trigger symptoms. Antacids, barbiturates, Tagamet, and iron and mineral supplements can prevent or reduce proper absorption of doxycycline. Like other antibiotics, this drug can create increased susceptibility to yeast infections and should be avoided in patients for whom this is a problem.

• Estrogen therapy: The suspicion that hormonal imbalances may worsen the symptoms of chronic fatigue syndrome has prompted some physicians to prescribe the sex hormone estrogen to female patients. Estrogen, which is traditionally used to alleviate menopausal symptoms, also relieves vaginitis and can produce a calming effect especially when prescribed in conjunction with mild tranquilizers. Common side effects of estrogen use include altered menstrual periods and yeast infections.

Several experimental therapies are also under scrutiny:

• Adenosine monophosphate (AMP): AMP, which eases joint and tendon inflammation and has proven effective against herpes virus infections, may also be useful in the treatment of chronic fatigue syndrome. Naturally occurring adenosine monophosphate enables cells to produce energy and to repair themselves; a viral infection depletes the body's supply of AMP, weakening the natural defense system. Preliminary reports indicate that intramuscular injections of AMP help build back the body's defense system, but the drug is not yet in common use and may currently be obtained only with special permission from the Food and Drug Administration.

• Kutapressin: Used primarily to reduce swelling and inflammation in certain skin disorders, including poison ivy, hives, acne, eczema, and severe sunburn, Kutapressin has also improved the overall health of a small sample of CFS patients. The drug is available only by injection and must be administered on a daily basis. Early but promising results need to be verified by other researchers.

• Transfer factor: This is a controversial therapy in which an ailing individual is injected with an extract obtained from the immune cells of someone who has recovered from the same disease. Records of attempts to transfer immunity from one person to another date back to World War II, with notable success in the treatment of hepatitis and tuberculosis. The availability of transfer factor is limited, however, and it is of little use in CFS until a specific immune deficiency is confirmed.

• Ampligen: An experimental drug purported to have immune-system-boosting capacities, ampligen is currently used only on an experimental basis with AIDS patients. A study of CFS patients is currently underway.

Self-Help Remedies That Work

Although it would be easy to entrust your doctor with full responsibility for your health care, it would not be wise. While your doctor can prescribe medications to relieve your symptoms and bolster your strength, ultimate control over life-style decisions and the capacity to cope rests in your hands. In this section, we'll discuss ways in which you can contribute to the painstaking process of rebuilding your health.

Sensitizing yourself to the reactions of your own body is an important first step. Learn what triggers your worst symptoms, how to avoid those triggers, and how to balance your need for rest with the importance of getting adequate exercise. You can also work to reduce the stress points in your life. While the precise role of stress in CFS remains a controversial and sensitive subject, it is known to exacerbate the symptoms of any chronic disease. "We tend to dismiss the fact that chronic stress has a physical effect on you," says Dr. Nathaniel Brown of North Shore University Hospital. "People can't cope until they stop denying that their own expectations are excessive or that they are stressed out. Recognizing your stressors goes a long way toward symptomatic relief." Stress reduction techniques, such as deep breathing, meditation, and biofeedback, can be enormously helpful.

Monitor Your Flare-Up Triggers

Sometimes there is an obvious reason for flaring symptoms: a stressful event, too much energetic activity, a cold, or the flu. Other triggers differ from one individual to another and are often unpredictable. Exposure to toxins such as auto exhaust, cigarette smoke, formaldehyde, household cleaning products, or other chemicals seems to make some people feel worse while others can't tolerate dust, molds, or pollen. High humidity, changes in the weather, or even exposure to sun and heat take their toll.

Right now we don't really understand why some people are

affected by certain triggers whereas others are not, but as a patient, it is important to figure out the progression of your own illness. Keeping a journal is one way to do so. Make notes on a daily basis about your health. Along with some general statements about the nature and severity of your symptoms, note the weather, your activities, the extent of your social interactions, what you have eaten, how much rest you have gotten, whether you are under pressure at work or at home, and if you have been knowingly exposed to pollutants or chemical toxins. If you are faithful about maintaining the journal, you may soon see a pattern emerge that will help you identify situations to avoid and provide some hints on what to do to keep your symptoms in check.

Rest, Rest, and More Rest

Although it is hard advice to swallow, the consensus among patients is that prolonged rest is the single most effective treatment available. "I hate to admit it but I feel best when I do almost nothing at all. It is when I try to be active that my symptoms flare," said a patient at a support group meeting in Charlotte, North Carolina.

Most people suffering from chronic fatigue syndrome function best if they sleep long hours—at least ten to twelve hours is often the norm. "It certainly shortens my day, but I find that within reason I can function almost normally if I get ten hours of sleep a night—and at least an hour's nap during the day as well," says one woman who is on the road to recovery after two long years of poor health.

When an upcoming event is likely to be stressful or tiring, many patients rest up for days in advance. The term *aggressive rest therapy* has been coined to describe rest intended to stave off future fatigue, rather than simply to combat the weariness of the moment. "This illness rules my life but it isn't going to ruin it," says Barbara Cote, age fifty-four, a British native who now lives in the Queens neighborhood of Whitestone. An avid dancer, she'll set aside two days in order to enjoy a single evening of pleasure. Before she and her husband can attend a dinner-dance, she spends the entire day in bed—and the following day is usually devoted to recuperation. Even then, she can't dance the lindy the way she once did. "We'll do a slow dance and as soon as I get hot and sweaty that will be my cue to stop. I'll sit down and hopefully later I'll get to do another slow dance. I just can't push myself. It's when you overstep that mark that the problems arise."

Do All Things in Moderation

Securing adequate rest works hand in glove with learning what your limits are—and respecting them. "I talk to people about life-style changes and about adapting," says Dr. Steven Marlowe, an infectious disease specialist in Atlanta. "I try to get people to think this thing through in terms of the Aristotelian mean, to moderate things. If they can avoid the deep valleys and high peaks, they can wind up better off and still accomplish wonderful things in their lives."

Whether or not you have been one of the superachievers who seems particularly susceptible to chronic fatigue syndrome, you will almost assuredly have to adjust your priorities and monitor your energies more carefully. Accustomed to jogging five miles every morning? Try to be satisfied with walking ten blocks instead. Were you a superaggressive salesperson? Perhaps you can develop some new sales techniques or content yourself with lesser achievements. "There are lots of concerts and movies I don't see, restaurants I don't eat at, exhibits I miss," acknowledged Lynn C., a forty-two-year-old Florida woman. "But I do go out every day. I make it a point to walk at least twenty blocks, which is sometimes the only exercise I get. I try to make the most out of the narrowed window of energy that I've got."

Like Lynn C., the patients who function best are those who come to accept this hard truth: To live well with chronic fatigue syndrome, you must turn down the rheostat of your life.

Take a Rational Approach
to Exercise

When dragging yourself from the bedroom to the bathroom is exhausting, you don't need to be reminded to cut back on your vigorous tennis game or to drop out of aerobics class. The athletic accomplishments that may once have been a source of pride to you are obviously out of the question for now. Remember, though, that total bed rest can be very deleterious to your health—after a few days, you lose vital nutrients, blood circulation is affected, and fewer gastric juices are secreted. To avoid further health problems, a minimum level of physical activity is recommended. Gentle stretching and slow walks are safe for almost everyone and help prevent muscle atrophy and maintain a minimal level of strength.

As your health begins to improve, you will probably be eager to begin a more rigorous exercise regimen, especially if you have been accustomed to regular workouts. Physicians urge extreme caution in doing so. For reasons that are not well understood, even modest exercise can produce a relapse. Seek a level of exercise that you can readily tolerate but bear in mind that a therapeutic level for one person can exhaust another or cause flaring discomfort.

Improve Your Eating Habits

Making appropriate dietary changes is one of the most concrete ways CFS patients can assert a degree of control over their health. The principles of sound nutrition are not radical ones. You don't have to switch to a macrobiotic diet or give up all red meats in order to eat more nutritionally. But helping your body work for you rather than against you, experimenting with what your system can tolerate, and learning to eat a balanced diet make good common sense. Consuming whole grains and beans while cutting back on fats, cholesterol, sodium, sugars, and meats that are hard to digest seems to help. Fresh fruits and vegetables are good, although some patients report digestive troubles, especially when raw foods are consumed late in the day. Even mild stimulants, such as coffee, alcohol, or nicotine, are generally ill-advised and sometimes intolerable to CFS patients.

"I used to mainline coffee just to get through the day," says Charles M., who has been sick for more than a year. "But I've weaned myself from all caffeine products and now I don't even drink a glass of wine. I try to eat mostly whole grains and very little meat. I just don't want to be consuming things that are going to put a strain on my body." Charles M.'s conscious efforts to maintain a healthy diet reap not only physiological rewards but psychic ones as well. "Given that there is no pill I can take for this thing, careful eating habits at least make me feel that I'm doing something to get well. There is an element of control here that is totally lacking in the rest of my life," he says.

Some patient groups recommend a visit to a hospital dietician, who can review your current diet and offer suggestions for improving it. Meanwhile, following are some dietary guidelines to help boost your general level of well-being:

- Avoid food with preservatives, dyes, or other chemical additives. Read the ingredient labels on any frozen, canned, or packaged foods you buy and check with your produce dealer before purchasing fruits and vegetables, which are often sprayed with sulfites to prevent rotting. Many states have now passed legislation requiring that signs be posted at salad bars when sulfites are used.

• Avoid alcohol. One of the peculiar hallmarks of chronic fatigue syndrome is an intolerance to liquor in any form. The use of caffeine, which is present not only in coffee but in tea, cola drinks, chocolate, and elsewhere, should also be heavily restricted.

• Cut back on refined sugars and avoid Nutrasweet, also known by its generic name, aspertame. Watch for hidden sources of sugar—it is often present in canned goods, prepared foods, and bread. Table sugar, honey, molasses, or corn syrup each provide an immediate surge of energy but then blood sugar crashes below its previous level, making you feel more tired than ever.

• Substitute herbs and spices for salt. Read product labels and you'll discover that breakfast cereals, many cheeses, most processed foods, cured meats, crackers, and many bread products are usually loaded with some form of sodium.

• Follow the dietary guidelines prescribed by the American Heart Association and restrict your consumption of fats to no more than 30 percent of your total caloric intake. Unsaturated fats, such as most vegetable oils, lower cholesterol level whereas saturated fats, including butter and meat fats, make it soar.

• Patients who tend to be gaseous or to suffer from an upset stomach should take added precautions. A good policy is to avoid solid foods for up to four hours before going to bed. A number of spices—including coriander seed, cloves, cumin seed, curry powder, mace, mustard powder, pepper, and cinnamon— can irritate the digestive tract. Certain raw fruits and vegetables, including broccoli, cauliflower, lettuce, and corn are also hard to digest and should be avoided if they pose a problem.

• Small but fairly frequent meals are easiest to digest and provide a somewhat more consistent level of energy to people with CFS.

Be Practical

CFS patients have stockpiled a warehouse of tricks to accomplish the basic chores of daily living while avoiding exhaustion. Some of these practical tips provide symptomatic relief while others help you channel precious energy so that you can function as normally as possible within the strict limitations of chronic illness. And this, in turn, can bolster your self-worth and provide an all-important sense of accomplishment.

- Get organized and plan ahead. Even if you do not have the flagging memory that is so characteristic of the syndrome, making lists is one way to avoid endless trips up and down a flight of stairs or getting back from the store only to discover that you have forgotten something crucial. Strategically placed sticky-pad notes can be an enormously helpful way of reminding you about what needs to get done.

- Try to schedule your errands at off-peak hours or during the times of the day when you are most energetic. Don't forget to dress warmly when going out. Better still, have a friend or neighbor shop for you at least occasionally.

- Prepare for a long day away from home by carrying any equipment that helps you function more easily. More than one patient has a story to tell about plopping down in the aisle of a store, overcome by exhaustion. An ingenious hint for avoiding embarrassment comes from a Chicago woman who carries a folding cane seat with her wherever she goes. Lightweight and easy to carry, she stores it in the back of her car and then transfers it to a shopping cart. Patients who do not ordinarily need canes often carry them when they expect to be out for many hours.

- Make it a point to sit down whenever possible. Most chores related to cooking and personal grooming can be done in a seated position.

- Dress comfortably in loose-fitting, easy-to-remove garments and have your hair done in an easy-to-manage style. Select easy-to-care-for fabrics to avoid extra laundering time. Wear shoes with little or no heel and be sure they provide good support.

- Avoid unnecessary stretching and bending, particularly if you have balance problems. Reorganize your kitchen, closets, and shelves so that frequently used items are within easy reach.

- Take advantage of mail-order and delivery services. With mail-order catalogs proliferating, and increasing numbers of stores and restaurants offering home-delivery services, especially in urban areas, chronically ill people need not want for many of life's comforts. On the other hand, don't neglect the importance of fresh air. Even if you can't walk a long distance, a brief foray outdoors helps clear your head.

• Plan simple and nourishing meals and always double or triple your recipes so that you can freeze the leftovers. Keep the pantry supplied with enough convenience foods to tide you over during the bad periods when the mere thought of leaving the house is exhausting.

• Along with improving the quality of your sleep, brief naps or deep meditation help ease throbbing pain and restore equilibrium. If you feel chilled upon awakening, consider the use of an electric blanket. Drinking hot liquids is another good way to counteract chills.

• Relieve numbing headaches with chemical cold and heat packs, which are more convenient and longer-lasting than traditional ice packs. Long hot soaks in the bathtub and a regular massage are good nonpharmaceutical ways to ease small discomforts that can add up to much misery. If a professional masseuse is not available in your community, consider swapping massages with a friend.

About Alternative Therapies

Skepticism toward the pharmaceutical and surgical bias of Western medicine did not begin with chronic fatigue syndrome. So-called alternative therapies, herbal remedies, and natural healing techniques have been used around the world for centuries. As the scientific community learns more about the mind–body connection, and understands the significance of time-honored healing practices, it is likely that many seemingly unconventional theories will grow in stature and acceptance. We have already seen this happen with the Chinese art of acupuncture, for example. Chiropractic treatment, too, has largely lost its image as a tool of charlatans and is now accorded due respect.

Unfortunately there is an accusatory strain within the holistic health movement suggesting that the fault for any sickness lies with the victim. This is not true, it's not fair, and it is not helpful. Clearly, a positive outlook on life, determination, and a passionate commitment to get well are tools for building good health that should not be lightly dismissed. But the claim that all ailing people have the capacity to heal themselves shows a remarkable ignorance of modern medicine and does a disservice to patients and physicians alike.

"It is important to view the mind–body connection in a nonpunitive way," says San Francisco social worker Ricki Boden, who has a special interest in counseling disabled persons. "To say that a psychological cure will effect a body cure is to say that you are to blame for your own illness. We just don't have that much control over the reality of disease."

The Appeal of Holistic Medicines

CFS patients feel that to a great extent they have been failed by Western medicine. Remarked New Jersey support group leader Bob Landau: "It is certainly possible that holistic medicine has something to offer us. Traditional medicine doesn't have a stranglehold on the truth."

Fortunately it is not necessary to forsake orthodox Western medicine practices entirely if you decide to learn about and experiment with unconventional therapies. While most Western doctors have not been formally trained in nutritional therapy and other techniques of natural healing, many respect their scientific validity. You don't need anyone's approval to pursue alternative treatment regimens, of course, but it is wise to keep your doctor informed and to heed warnings about hazardous practices.

San Francisco internist Neil Singer takes a fairly unconventional stance toward many holistic remedies. While cautioning that each one must be considered individually—and with a rather large grain of salt—he is perfectly willing to have his patients try such products as germanium and coenzyme Q12, which are alleged to boost the immune system. "These can't hurt and some of my patients tell me they got better," notes Singer. "Those who push these things have theoretical reasons for why they work and they make some sense." Along with a traditional treatment regimen, Singer therefore listens closely when patients describe their use of alternative remedies and passes along any information he gleans to others who ask for it.

Healthy skepticism, however, is the order of the day when considering nontraditional approaches. Frantic for a cure, CFS patients are easy prey to the con artists and snake doctors who peddle worthless formulas to the gullible. One local support group leader warns: "There are so many bizarre treatments being recommended today. And there are a lot of people willing to make a fast buck off a new, mysterious illness." One patient has been heard discussing the healing powers of super blue-green algae and another swears that being hooked up to a generator and jolted with electricity is the best cure for the syndrome. "If someone tells me the solution is fish oil capsules, heck, I'll try fish oil capsules," admits an actor who has suffered the pain of chronic fatigue syndrome for five years. "After what I have been through, I figure anything is worth a try."

Understandable, perhaps, but the consequences of that attitude can be devastating. No error is more serious than believing that a treatment is harmless merely because it is labeled "alternative." Sheer desperation should never be allowed to supplant good judgment.

A Sampler of Therapies

Deep relaxation techniques, meditation, and yoga have been praised for their capacity to relieve chronic pain and to counter the physical manifestations of stress. Nutritional supplements, including megadoses of vitamins, herbs, bee pollen, and numerous plant extracts have also received attention, as have countless other products sold in most health food stores. Although none is certain to cure what ails you, each of the techniques described here has provided relief to some chronic fatigue syndrome patients. Volumes have been written on these and many other therapies and interested patients should refer to Appendix C for sources of more detailed information on holistic healing.

Nutritional Therapy. Nutritional science is a subject far too complex to probe here, but a few vitamins, minerals, and plant extracts are worth mentioning. Of particular interest to CFS patients are vitamins A, B_6, B_{12}, C, and E, as well as zinc, folic acid, and selenium, all of which are said to have immune-boosting potential. The minerals folic acid and lysine may have some capacity to counteract the effect of herpes viruses. Germanium, a popular herbal remedy that is found naturally in garlic, ginseng, and comfrey, is being investigated by the Food and Drug Administration for its potential to bolster immune system function. Lomatrium, a plant that grows at high elevations in the United States and Canada and has been used by American Indians for centuries to combat colds and pneumonia, is also attracting interest. Chinese herbal remedies have reportedly relieved symptomatic discomfort, and a number of patients swear by Sunrider Chinese herbs.

Oil extract from the seeds of the evening primrose plant is another medicine of the American Indians and some CFS patients have also experimented with this natural remedy. The evening primrose plant is distinguished by its bright yellow flowers and grows wild along the roadside and in sand dunes. The theoretical basis for its use is that evening primrose oil contains gamma-linolenic acid (GLA), which converts in the body to prostaglandin, a vital substance in the regulation of cellular function. Unfortunately, there has been little scientific investigation into any of these nutritional therapies.

Homeopathy. Practiced both by well-trained lay persons and by a small number of physicians, homeopathy is based on the theory that like cures like. Curiously it was developed at the end of the eighteenth century in Leipzig, Germany by Dr. Samuel Hahnemann at virtually the same moment that Edward Jenner was developing the world's first vaccine, predicated on much the same principle.

Homeopaths are more interested in the symptoms of a disease than in its cause, making this avenue of alternative medicine particularly appropriate for CFS patients. Once a homeopath understands the precise nature of your symptoms, tiny, highly diluted doses of a medicine that ordinarily *causes* these symptoms is administered. The underlying principle of homeopathy is that symptoms are a signal of the body's efforts to cure itself and remedies that cause similar effects stimulate the immune system to do its job more effectively.

Biofeedback. An art that has gained a great deal of respect among orthodox practitioners in recent years, biofeedback provides a palpable measurement of the mind–body connection. By monitoring physiological changes with a hand temperature meter, an electrical skin resistance meter, or an electromyograph, which measures muscular activity, biofeedback alerts individuals to sources of stress and its manifestations. Relaxation techniques, counseling, or other medical or holistic therapies are generally used in conjunction with biofeedback to help individuals control the nervous system functions that were once thought to be entirely automatic.

Visualization Therapy. An ancient healing technique still used in certain Eskimo and Indian cultures, visualization is thought to be a powerful tool for focusing and activating mental energy. With the help of a trained therapist, patients learn to visualize a scene that allows them to feel pleasure, to relax more deeply, to imagine the healing process taking place, or to witness obstacles to good health being removed.

A cancer patient, for example, might envision cancerous cells being consumed by healthy cells; an automobile accident victim might picture the healing of broken bones. CFS patients can visualize themselves as wholly well and functioning people, can picture inflammation going down, or can turn the mind's eye toward a mental battle between fatigue and energy, with energy emerging triumphant.

Reflexology. Although it has been an ancient art in Asia, Western reflexology has been developed only during the twentieth century. Practitioners say that zones in the feet and hands correspond to certain body organs, and that by external massage, manipulation, and pressure, the functioning of internal organs can be improved. Because it can induce a state of deep relaxation, reflexology is particularly effective when used to relieve pain.

Final Words of Caution

Regardless of the combination of medications, holistic remedies, self-care, and lifestyle adaptation that works best for you, a number of obstacles present themselves along the road to recovery. Three warnings are particularly appropriate: Don't exchange information with other patients too casually, beware of the risks of substance abuse, and take steps to protect your health as you begin to recover.

The Perils of Exchanging Information

In the absence of a magic bullet to cure you, and with so much uncertainty surrounding effective treatments, patients tend to compare notes on the prescription drugs, over-the-counter medications, holistic remedies, and vitamin regimens they are trying. Although the intention is benign, an alarming amount of inaccurate or even dangerous information can be passed along by doing so. Remember that one person's medicine might be another's poison. Someone might have an allergic reaction to a medication that has worked for you. Another might advocate a "miracle cure" when in fact he simply went into spontaneous remission for no obvious reason. And patients rarely know the risks of drug interactions or the likelihood that certain combinations of over-the-counter and prescription drugs can cumulatively weaken or intensify the effects of each medication.

Talking to other patients is fine but the only safe rule of thumb is to take no medication without a doctor's knowledge.

Beware of Substance Abuse

Anyone with a chronic illness is at higher risk for substance abuse, and as a patient, or as a friend or family member, you should remain alert to this possibility. The problem is heightened with CFS because doctors can do so little to cure it and may be tempted to overmedicate. Commonly prescribed painkillers, tranquilizers, and sleeping pills can be readily abused, especially if a patient sees more than one doctor. Be sure to bring your medication log to medical appointments to remind your doctor of your current prescriptions.

As with any patient population, there will also be people who deal with the frustration, anger, and fear of chronic illness by turning to the mind-numbing drugs that make it possible to forget pain and uncertainty. Patients may also be tempted to experiment with home remedies, over-the-counter medications, and illegal drugs, any of which can be very potent indeed. While most physicians routinely monitor the use of prescription drugs, they often fail to inquire about other self-medicating regimens.

Stay alert to the very real dangers of substance abuse and seek medical advice or psychological counseling if you find you are becoming dependent on certain drugs.

Safeguard Your Recovery

The curative powers of time, coupled with some of the treatment regimens described here, are likely to move you slowly toward improved health. But CFS patients may still need to take special precautions for many years. You can guard against relapse and ensure a long-lasting recovery by staying attuned to your body and responding quickly to the first sign of recurrent symptoms. If certain medications have been effective, discontinue them only under physician guidance. Maintain the eating and sleeping habits that helped relieve your symptoms and continue to exercise caution before assuming new commitments. Above all, don't be too hasty to return to the routines of yesteryear's stress-filled life: Remember, stress may well have contributed to your illness in the first place.

Along with the struggle to find appropriate medical care and treatments that work, you will probably have a lot to do to put your emotional and financial house in order. Enduring a chronic illness can mean coping with a shattered ego, learning to communicate in new ways with loved ones, and dealing with friends who don't know what to say and family members who are not sure how to help. It can also mean cutting back on job-related responsibilities, accepting career limitations, and sometimes losing a hard-won position.

In the next part of this book, we'll focus on the emotional and financial issues raised by chronic fatigue syndrome. First, though, let's meet briefly with some of the top-level physicians involved in CFS research and treatment.

Profiles: The Physicians

Today chronic fatigue syndrome has earned a place on the nation's health agenda, but in the mid-1980s, the few physicians and researchers working in the field labored in obscurity and isolation. Some were scoffed at; others were advised to switch fields or suffer the consequences of a damaged professional reputation. Instead they persevered and went on to become leaders in the growing field of CFS research.

Here are portraits of some of these pioneers. Also included in this section is a look at a conference held in Newport, Rhode Island, which brought together major researchers and patient leaders from all over the country.

Dr. Paul Cheney
Nalle Clinic: Charlotte, North Carolina

Since 1984, when his private practice in Incline Village, Nevada was inundated by a CFS epidemic of startling proportions, Dr. Paul Cheney has lectured and written widely about the syndrome, poured his own resources into research, and treated patients who traveled hundreds or thousands of miles to seek his guidance. The maverick internist is something of a legend among chronic fatigue syndrome patients. "He laid his professional reputation on the line for us," says one patient, citing Cheney's willingness to buck a skeptical medical establishment in order to bring public attention to the mystifying illness.

Speaking from his offices at the Nalle Clinic in Charlotte, North Carolina, where he now practices, the intense, soft-spoken physician explains why he does not doubt for a moment that CFS is a genuine problem with organic origins.

> It is the patients who are clearly ill and clearly have so little to gain by being ill who become our beacons in the night. All physicians who come to believe in this have had two or more of these people who convince them that it is real. If you see someone with a lot of psychological overlay, someone with a lot of secondary gain, then I'd be skeptical too, but if you see someone who is as well as you and I and they just get *crushed* by this, you become a believer.

Almost alone among his colleagues, Cheney suspects chronic fatigue syndrome represents a distinct new problem.

I have never seen anything like this in my whole life. All of a sudden these people are coming out of the woodwork. Isn't it strange that in the twentieth century, with a disease this impressive to look at, we have such a poor idea about what it is? I think that's because there is something new out there."

Cheney approaches CFS as an intellectual puzzle, calling it "the most fascinating thing I've ever seen." As he talks about the potentially calamitous consequences of CFS, Cheney broods aloud about the extinction of species and the possibility that the dinosaurs were obliterated by an unknown microorganism. He's not exactly suggesting that CFS could do the same thing to human beings but he's fearful about the evolution of virulent new viruses. "You have to wonder what the hell is going on here. First you have AIDS, then chronic fatigue syndrome, what else is coming down the pike?"

Cheney takes a conciliatory stance toward the disagreements that divide the scientific community. In his ideal world, those who view CFS skeptically will listen and learn from the converted while the converts will study the viewpoint of the skeptics.

With this disease, up is down and down is up, so you need to be very subtle in your thinking. The worst thing a physician can be is dogmatic. That's why even examining the perspectives of critics who doubt that the whole thing exists is worthwhile because there must be something here that makes them think that. Most likely, neither of us is totally wrong or totally right but we can each learn from the other.

Dr. Stephen Straus
National Institute of Allergy and Infectious Diseases: Bethesda, Maryland

Dr. Stephen Straus's research into chronic fatigue syndrome dates back to 1985, when he was the leading author of a now-famous article suggesting an association between the Epstein-Barr virus and chronic illness in adults. A leading medical virologist at the National Institute of Allergy and Infectious Diseases, a branch of the National Institutes of Health, Dr. Straus continues to publish widely on the subject of chronic fatigue syndrome and is following some 150 patients over a period of years to monitor the course of their disease.

In a cubicle office in legendary Building Ten—said to be the largest brick structure on earth—on the verdant Maryland campus of the National Institutes of Health, Straus talked about the uncertainty of chronic fatigue syndrome and its impact on patients.

There is a difference between people who have this syndrome and people who have other chronic illnesses that can't be treated in a specific way. Other patients at least know what to expect from their disease and everyone believes them. CFS patients don't know what to expect and not everyone believes them. That's why these patients actually need and demand more from their doctors even though their disease is not progressive or life-threatening.

Somewhat acerbic in manner, Straus has raised the hackles of some CFS patients with his frank discussion of the link between chronic fatigue syndrome and depression. Referring to findings of immune system abnormalities in CFS patients, Straus notes:

If one reads the psychiatric literature, one can see many of the same differences from the norm. And studies dating back to the 1940s, 1950s and early 1960s show that individuals who take a long time to recover from certain infections have a different psychological makeup than those who do not.

Despite the controversial implications of his statements, Straus says, "All the symptoms that these patients have are symptoms that all of us have had on some occasion," noting that this fact substantiates the credibility of CFS in his mind. "To say that there are mechanisms within all of us that make us feel the same way for a short period of time suggests that these very same mechanisms could be persistent in a smaller population group."

The raging debate about the true nature of chronic fatigue syndrome can only be put to rest with an analysis of carefully compiled data, insists Straus, noting that "blind men view the elephant very differently. One has to be open to the possibility that this is constructed very differently than one's first impression leads one to imagine."

Dr. Carol Jessop
Fairmount Medical Group: El Cerrito, California

While medical researchers argue the fine points of causality and debate rages over the merits of allocating public funds to CFS, primary-care physicians are struggling to care for the countless thousands of frightened and hurting patients who need help. Dr. Carol Jessop is one of this dedicated breed.

A specialist in women's health care, Jessop was affiliated with the University of California at San Francisco and working part-time in a community clinic when she was introduced to chronic fatigue syndrome in 1983. Within a four-month period, she had seen three patients who were complaining of extraordinary fatigue. "All day long I hear people come in and say they are tired. But this was qualitatively different," recalls Jessop. "These people were describing a fatigue so devastating they could not get out of bed."

Along with an exhaustion that drastically slowed the tempo of their lives, Jessop's patients described aches and nausea, a tendency to fall toward one side while walking, and terrible sleep disorders. "It was clear to me that none of the three were depressed," says Jessop, noting that she regularly diagnoses and treats classic depression. After taking careful histories and listening to a description of their symptoms, Dr. Jessop recalls telling each one: "Well, it sounds like you either have an infection or an autoimmune disease. I don't think it is cancer because you are a young, healthy person, but that would be third on my list. Now, let's go to work."

After extensive laboratory tests and consultations with specialists revealed nothing extraordinary, Jessop could offer those early patients little more than symptomatic relief. But unlike some physicians, who grow discouraged and skeptical at that point, Jessop found herself drawn further into the detective story of CFS. Within two years of treating her first patients, sixty more had made their way to her office. Word traveled that Jessop was responsive and concerned, and by 1988, another six hundred had sought her help. By then she had moved into the East Bay offices of the Fairmount Medical Group, a forty-five-minute train ride from San Francisco. Frightened chronic fatigue syndrome patients continued to pound at her door, eventually forcing her to restrict her practice and refer the overflow elsewhere.

Jessop is less sanguine than many of her colleagues about the course and long-term consequences of CFS.

> After following patients for five years, I am terribly concerned about sequelae with this illness, which includes central nervous system disease as well as thyroid disease and some endocrine problems. I don't know how it is transmitted; I don't know what to tell patients about contagiousness. I am trying various things, like my colleagues are. And I feel overwhelmed by the illness.

Ultimately, though, Jessop is convinced CFS will command attention. "It is getting to the point where most people know someone who has this illness and that's when things start to move. As soon as famous people are affected, everyone will learn about the syndrome."

Medical Conference, Newport, Rhode Island

Newport, Rhode Island is better known for its yachts and mansions than for its medical conferences, but a rainy weekend's event at the city's Marriott Hotel may help change this perception. Several hundred researchers, physicians, support group leaders, and patients recently gathered at the Marriott on America's Cup Avenue to discuss CFS, to exchange theories about cause and treatment, to describe ongoing research, and to send a message of hope to all who suffer.

The conference was cosponsored by the Rhode Island General Assembly, the state Department of Health, and the Brown University Program in Medicine; the list of participants reads like a *Who's Who* in chronic fatigue syndrome. Among the panelists were Dr. Anthony Komaroff, Brigham and Women's Hospital, Boston, Massachusetts; Dr. James F. Jones, National Jewish Center for Immunology and Respiratory Medicine, Denver, Colorado; Dr. Paul R. Cheney, Nalle Clinic, Charlotte, North Carolina; and Dr. Robert Hallowitz, private practice, Gaithersburg, Maryland. Top political leaders, including Governor Edward D. DiPrete, U.S. Senator Claiborne Pell, and U.S. Representative Claudine C. Schneider, also spoke briefly. Representatives from the National Institutes of Health, the Centers for Disease Control, the Social Security Administration, and university and medical laboratories around the country were in the audience.

Dr. H. Denman Scott, Director of Rhode Island's Department of Health, opened the conference by saying, "It's about time we get serious about a problem that has affected many of our citizens, leaving them going from pillar to post, wondering whether they are crazy or their doctors are crazy." Dr. Scott then asked panelists to describe their own findings, speculate about cause, exchange ideas on treatment, and answer questions from the audience.

Dr. James Jones described several key CFS research projects underway in Denver—notably, a study of immune system abnormalities, a look at the genetic propensity for illness, and refinements in the definition of CFS. Better ways to measure syndrome symptoms should also be a research priority, according to Dr. Anthony Komaroff. "We need to compare measurements in CFS with people feeling perfectly healthy and also with those who have pure depressive disorders," said Komaroff, noting that such comparisons will enable physicians to pinpoint the abnormalities that specifically characterize chronic fatigue syndrome.

While acknowledging the importance of ongoing research, Dr. Robert Hallowitz urged that appropriate treatment for CFS be made a priority, noting "While we wait for specific research to be completed, we have to deal with the fact that many people are going down the tubes." If AIDS is a death sentence, CFS is a life sentence, said Hallowitz, urging physicians to emphasize ways to give patients a renewed sense of control over their destinies.

At a fund-raising event sponsored by the CFIDS Association and targeted at Washington, D.C. lobbying activities, Dr. David Bell, the Lyndonville, New York pediatrician, talked about the devastating consequences of CFS on children and adolescents. Isolated from friends, unable to participate in sports or family activities, and often labeled school phobic, they may suffer even more than adults, who are generally more secure in their identities. "Adolescence is a crucial time of development. Someone who misses six months or more of school may develop problems that will last a lifetime," Bell said somberly.

The interest of the medical and public health communities that was so visible at the Newport conference augurs well for a commitment to a cure. In summing up the day's events, Komaroff urged physicians to "leave today believing this is an illness to be taken seriously," and he told patients:

> I hope you are as impressed as we are by what has happened with this illness in the past four years. Four years ago those of you who were suffering from this illness and those of us who were beginning to work on it were really pretty much alone. That has changed. It hasn't changed enough and it hasn't changed fast enough. But when I consider how different things are today, how many thousands are across the world discussing this illness, and how much increased emphasis there has been in the last year on supporting research, I find the state of things very encouraging. I hope you share that conviction.

PART III

Learning to
Cope

6

.

Staying Centered:
Tools for Emotional
Survival

There is one thing I think about almost every day that helps me get
through, especially when the going is particularly rough. It is this
quote from Nietzsche: "What does not destroy me, makes me
stronger." And this serves always to remind me how something good
will arise from the ashes of my own suffering.

—Condy Eckerle, age twenty-five,
CFS patient, New York, New York

I don't choose to be called a victim of chronic fatigue syndrome. I
prefer to call myself a survivor.

—Linda Dooley, CFS support group
leader, Providence, Rhode Island

The news that they may remain ill for months or years is devastating
to an accomplished and productive population accustomed to a lifetime
of good health. Patients have likened their sense of loss and confusion
to that of a sailor marooned at sea. As he is without moorings, they are
without the comforting familiarity of daily routine, and both drift
steadily away from safe harbor.

In the grip of chronic fatigue syndrome, patients have no option
but to curtail their activities drastically, a change of pace that requires
tremendous psychological adjustment. Bedridden patients must learn
to cope with isolation, boredom, and an exhaustion that twelve hours
of sleep fails to cure. Painstakingly laid plans and aspirations often
turn overnight to dust and the realities of aging and human mortality

strike with the force of a ton of bricks. Meanwhile, the terms of personal relationships, most likely established in the pink of health, must be renegotiated. Sometimes the bonds of love and friendship cannot tolerate the strain of change and are severed.

The workplace offers no greater protection. Those who have defined themselves as working professionals may find their sense of identity shattered. A Wall Street trader is suddenly unable to balance her own checkbook. A superwoman who once so successfully juggled career and family becomes overwhelmed at the complexities of sorting the silverware as she empties the dishwasher. The prospect of losing a job suddenly looms large, fueling a sense of vulnerability, the threat of a financial crisis, and the sensation that life is spiraling out of control.

To this ordeal, add the skepticism that still nips at the heels of chronic fatigue syndrome patients, and the package of misery is complete. One patient had to deal so often with the accusation that she was a hypochondriac that when she was also diagnosed with cancer she recalls a feeling of relief. "Cancer, at least, is something that people understand and can sympathize with," she said.

No wonder, then, that chronic fatigue syndrome places an enormous emotional strain on its targets. And yet for every tale told of hardship and suffering there is another about courage and resilience. Deep inside all of us lie untapped reserves of strength that can become a life-sustaining force in times of physical and emotional pain. The CFS patients who cope most effectively learn to harness those hidden reserves: Their trial by fire is arduous and they do not emerge unscarred, but they do adjust and they do survive. Some do so with the help of support groups; others find their answers in private or group therapy. Still others eschew formal support but master the survival tactics that enable them to survive the emotional devastation of chronic fatigue syndrome.

In this chapter, we'll look first at the emotional consequences of having a chronic illness and then discuss some of the tools for emotional survival.

The Emotional Impact of Chronic Illness

Sickness has been called an insult to the body but it is also a tremendous affront to the mind and to the spirit. Rare is the individual who can adjust to the trauma of chronic fatigue syndrome without first enduring a period of desperation. For some people, the worst moments come before diagnosis, in the days when an overactive imagination encourages fears of the worst. For others, the bleakest period follows diagnosis, when the reality of living with an unpredictable, long-term illness begins to sink in.

Chester Helms knows what desperation is all about—and he's something of an expert on overcoming obstacles as well. Thin and pale, Helms has been confined to a wheelchair since he broke his neck diving into a lake at age nineteen. Nonetheless, as head of Programs for Accessible Living (PAL) in Charlotte, North Carolina, he is a dynamic public speaker and a mover and shaker in local efforts to obtain rights for the disabled. PAL, which helps people cope with limited function, is collaborating with the Chronic Fatigue and Immune Dysfunction Syndrome (CFIDS) Association of North Carolina to make assistance to chronic fatigue syndrome patients a special priority. "You go down and down and you reach a point when you'll decide 'that's as far down as I can go and still maintain my sanity.' And that's when you really begin the struggle to cope," he told a support group recently.

Before CFS patients can truly come to grips with the physical and emotional consequences of their illness—and move on to rebuild their lives—they must first grieve for what has been lost.

The Grieving Process

In *On Death and Dying,* Elizabeth Kubler-Ross defines five stages through which bereaved individuals typically pass in the process of grieving for the loss of a loved one: denial, anger, bargaining, depression, and acceptance. An ailing patient, mourning for the bygone days of good health, goes through much the same ordeal.

Denial, a sort of mental numbness, comes first. Mustering all the forces of a strong defense mechanism, a patient declares that the doctors are wrong and insists the symptoms will not prove to be chronic in nature.

But it doesn't work: The symptoms do persist and frustration boils into anger. "How can this possibly happen to me?" a patient demands to know. "I've got so many plans for the future." An overpowering rage at life's unfairness impedes rational behavior. Friends and family are likely to come in for an unfair dosage of abuse during this stage.

In time, the anger dissipates and the deal making begins. During the bargaining stage, a patient decides that a cure can be effected with good intentions and determination. Wild promises often get made: "If I can just get well again, I'll always eat a healthy diet or slow down the tempo of my life or spend more time with my parents," pledge the patients as they dash madly from one specialist to another.

But no one keeps the other end of the patient's bargain and depression finally sets in. This is the penultimate stage of grief and it can be overwhelming. Suicidal thoughts, a paralysis of will, extreme guilt, severely disrupted eating and sleeping patterns, sexual dysfunction, and severe self-image problems are typical signals of depression.

The process is not entirely linear and patients can get stuck in any stage of grief, but the road is rockiest until they reach the acceptance stage. By acknowledging the reality of illness and its concomitant limitations, they can begin to adjust and adapt. "There is a need to come to terms with the illness and learn to live with it," says patient leader Bob Landau. "Many people are convinced this is the worst thing ever to happen to them but the bottom line is CFS is something we just have to learn to live with."

With acceptance comes an end to the frenetic odyssey through the health care system. Instead of trying every drug regimen and vitamin therapy that comes along, patients grow more skeptical and cautious. While remaining open to new therapies, they also accept the odds against a miracle cure. In the ensuing mood of greater tranquility, they begin at last to rebuild their self-esteem, and with it, their hopes and dreams for the future. Ultimately chronic fatigue syndrome becomes a background fact of life, not a foreground obsession.

That Desperate Moment: When Suicide Beckons

Bumping along the rocky road heading toward acceptance, more than one CFS patient has confessed that suicide—and the accompanying freedom from the burdens of chronic illness—sometimes seems tempting. "It's hard bucking illness and disbelief every day," said one woman. "You begin to feel very little desire to continue. I know that I have gone to bed thinking seriously, 'please God, let me go to sleep and just not wake up in the morning.' "

No matter how idly expressed, a suicide threat is at once a fantasy of liberation and a desperate cry for help, and it should never be dismissed lightly. Although the moment of blackness usually passes quickly, some 30,000 Americans die by their own hand every year. Depression, social isolation, and the loss of personal control greatly enhance the likelihood of suicide. Particularly at risk are individuals who tend to be impulsive, acting first, thinking later. Taking an overdose of drugs, for example, may be intended as a means to gain fast relief, not as a way to commit suicide—but by the time that realization hits, it can be too late. Drinking is definitely not recommended for suicidal individuals because it tends to loosen inhibitions and is a depressant.

Anyone who has recurrent or vivid thoughts of suicide should not delay in seeking help. Suicide hotlines have been established in most communities and professional counseling may also be in order. Crisis intervention can provide an immediate outlet for expressing fear and anger and help overcome feelings of desperation and helplessness. In the long run, skilled counseling can help suicidal individuals gain some perspective on their problems and return them to a life-sustaining sense of control.

Change, Not Transformation

While the emotional roller coaster of chronic fatigue syndrome eventually levels, coping with the stresses of a long-term illness is an ongoing process. Reactions necessarily mirror other attitudes in life. According to Ricki Boden, a licensed clinical social worker who counsels patients in San Francisco:

> Everyone brings to this illness what they are in the rest of their lives. A person who is obsessive at other times will be looking at every book and article written on the subject of chronic fatigue syndrome and seeing every doctor available. Someone who is inclined toward denial will pretend not to notice the sickness. A person who often becomes emotionally distraught will cope with the illness in the same way. CFS won't "metamorphosize" you.

But if an individual's core personality does not change, virtually every other aspect of life does. As competent, independent, and assertive adults lose their highly prized strength, self-image can take a terrible battering. Your world shrinks and the competitive pace of life beyond the security of home can seem overwhelming. "Once I loved to explore the city," said Mary A. "Now I find the streets too crowded. Everyone is moving very fast and talking very fast. I don't feel like I can keep up anymore."

At some point, CFS patients inevitably begin to compare themselves to their halcyon and able-bodied days, which can fuel a sense of hopelessness and depression. "This body is not the body I once had," wailed one woman. Jan Montgomery, a political organizer accustomed to meeting regularly with high-level public officials in San Francisco, says that when she became ill with CFS, she was initially unable to cope with such pressured meetings. "How could I meet with city supervisors? There were days I couldn't even meet the UPS man at the door."

Undergoing the rigors of chronic illness either breaks your spirits or deepens your determination, thinks Condy Eckerle, a Brooklyn patient, who says, "If it doesn't break you, being put in adverse conditions can have the opposite effect, bringing out your depth of understanding about larger truths and helping you overcome obstacles."

The Role of Support Groups

Some 400 support groups have been created in small towns and big cities across the country and around the world, mostly as a result of grassroots organizing by patients themselves. The growing network provides crucial emotional and practical help to countless thousands. No two support groups are exactly the same, with each setting an agenda to meet the particular needs and problems of its own community. The work generally falls into three interlinked areas:

- Informing and educating the general public, and particularly patients, their families, and the medical community.

- Counseling and consoling those who have been diagnosed with chronic fatigue syndrome.

- Organizing and advocating for the cause at both the local and the national level.

Is a Support Group for Me?

If you are a chronic fatigue syndrome patient—or if you love someone who is—joining a support group can be an empowering tool to help you regain control over your life. No matter how satisfied you are with your health care, it is unlikely that your doctors provide much emotional support—it isn't their job to do so, yet healing the mind is as important in the proper treatment of CFS as healing the body. Peer support is an indispensable complement to good medical care.

Some patients join a group when they are first diagnosed and need to learn more about their illness or cope with anger and confusion. Others, who have traveled further along the path toward recovery, may talk about their journey and provide straight-from-the-heart, I've-been-there-too encouragement. "I guess misery loves company but there's more going on here than that," said Mary A., who admitted she had never fully acknowledged the reality of her illness until attending her first support group meeting. "It helps to hear other people's personal stories and to know that it is normal to feel anxious and upset."

At the best support group meetings, you'll get up-to-the-minute information about the research progress being made on CFS as scientists and physicians search for a cause, experiment with new treatments, and work toward a cure. Many groups circulate articles from both the popular and scientific press and bring in experts to discuss their latest findings. You can also learn about the health care facilities available in your area. Physician referral lists are commonly maintained and many groups also compile detailed information from patients about the efficacy of their treatment and the compassion with which it has been dispensed.

Most important, you'll meet people who understand what you are going through and can remind you that you are not alone. A similar story is told over and again about patients attending their first support group meeting: When they meet their comrades-in-suffering and hear stories that are so much like their own, tears of relief flow fast and furiously. In an environment where the right to privacy is considered sacred, it is safe to cry and acceptable to ask for emotional support. For patients who have been isolated by illness, support groups fill a critical social function. They can be especially important for those without an extended network of friends and family living nearby.

Dropping In on a Meeting

They've been called "lifesavers" by grateful fans and "pity parties" by cynical detractors. But what really goes on at a support group meeting?

The setting is the spacious auditorium of Beth Israel Hospital in New York City. Fifty chronic fatigue syndrome patients—men and women, old and young—have come together to listen to a medical lecture and then to meet in small groups to share their personal experiences.

This month's speaker is Sharon Kaplan, a social worker who counsels chronic fatigue syndrome patients as part of a health care team at New York's Mount Sinai Hospital. Kaplan begins her talk by discussing theories of healing that date back to the Greeks. "Greek wisdom focused on the innate capacity of human beings to recover from illness and on the drive for wellness that is at the center of our beings. Physician intervention should foster those natural tendencies, not work against them," says Kaplan.

Noting that ancient societies have always believed the harmonious integration of our emotions, our thoughts, and our behavior to be crucial to good health, she adds, "With modern technology, perhaps we have turned our backs on something of great healing value. These are not mystical ideas, they have been time-honored across many cultures."

The social worker then speaks directly to the frustrations and anger felt by many CFS patients, acknowledging that patients often must deal with emotions they've never experienced before. "Who can have this condition without grief?" she asks. "While chronic fatigue syndrome isn't terminal, you are likely to feel that a great deal of your life has been taken from you."

Emphasizing the importance of relaxation to healing, Kaplan concludes her talk by guiding the group through a series of exercises intended to introduce them to meditation and deep breathing. Her presentation is followed by a question and answer session, and then the support group leader, a vibrant woman who endured the vagaries of chronic fatigue syndrome for six years, asks everyone to gather in a wagon-train circle.

Emotions are raw as each person speaks briefly about his or her own experiences. There is a haunting similarity to the stories—years of illness, misdiagnoses, skepticism from family members, thoughts of suicide, and from some, signs that they are finally back on the path to good health.

One young man says, "I'm gay and when I first started feeling sick I was sure I had AIDS. I was scared to death."

"I don't trust doctors anymore," says another patient, to sympathetic nods from others in the group. A nurse now on a leave of absence from her jobs says, "I feel fragile, feeble at times. I can't think, I can't concentrate, and I'm sleeping twelve to fourteen hours a day."

"Can't anyone help me?" pleads an elderly women desperately, the tears shining in her eyes. With that, the tone shifts to a more practical one. People describe their symptoms in clinical detail and get advice from others. They name doctors in the area who have been helpful and those who should be avoided at all costs. Diet and vitamin therapies are discussed along with the range of holistic and traditional treatment regimens. Given a medical establishment that has been able to do little for them, many concur with the woman who says, "Question your doctor's authority. Find out what is being prescribed for you and why."

Consult Appendix B in the back of the book for help in finding a support group in your community.

The Benefits of
Psychological Counseling

Skepticism and doubt about chronic fatigue syndrome have discouraged some individuals from seeking psychological counseling. The scars from friends and family who have hinted that CFS is more a disease of the mind than the body have not healed. Patients have gagged too many times on the bitter pills of doubt dispensed by their physicians and have heard too much careless talk about psychosomatic illness. Unwilling to fuel the suspicion that CFS is solely the manifestation of depression, they refuse the counseling that could make coping easier.

But any kind of chronic illness requires enormous psychic adjustment and appropriate therapy can play a crucial role in easing that adjustment. The mere fact of having a chronic illness that is poorly understood, cannot be effectively treated, and lingers for months or years is enough to make anyone depressed. "If you talk about the merits of psychotherapy, patients feel you are saying the illness is all in their heads," says a support group leader in Denver. "But every chronic illness has a psychological component to it. If it isn't there when you first get sick, it will develop somewhere along the way."

Making the very personal decision to seek professional help can be an act of courage, not an acknowledgment of defeat. It can be a way of saying, "I *will* survive the devastation of this illness but I need some help to do it." It can be a key to unlock the doors that have barred communication with loved ones and a tool to ask for what you need from them. Therapy can also provide an opportunity to vent feelings of rage for having been robbed of years of good health—and provide a means of moving past that rage to a place of peace.

Dr. Leonard Zegans, professor of psychiatry at the University of California at San Francisco, believes that consultation with a therapist can be enormously helpful to chronic fatigue syndrome patients. Zegans, who is involved in ground-breaking research to unravel the connection between an individual's psychological state and the reactivation of latent viruses, notes that a therapist can:

- Make a full assessment of a patient's stress level and capacity to cope. Regardless of what initially triggers a health problem, stress can impede recovery and interfere with the adjustment process. The intervention of a skillful therapist can have tangible payoffs in the form of physiological and psychological improvement.

- Evaluate a patient's available social support system and determine the extent to which family, friends, and work colleagues are understanding and supportive. A therapist can also work to educate family members about the illness and help them understand its consequences.

- Assess the impact of CFS on a patient's self-image. The loss of function, strength, or mental acuity can shatter an individual's confidence, which leads in turn to frustration or depression. Professional guidance may be needed to help patients come to grips with their own limitations and accept a redefined sense of self.

- Provide practical guidance in structuring daily activities to achieve maximum efficiency. For example, by identifying a patient's periods of optimum alertness, a therapist can help structure the day so that necessary projects get done.

"Therapy is enormously helpful to me in terms of getting regular emotional support," admits one patient, who must take a taxicab to her therapist's office just a few blocks away because she is too incapacitated to walk. "I get a lot of hand-holding and lots of nurturance and of course the human contact is so important. When you are sick, your life shrinks. The struggle now is just to get through every day and in therapy we deal constantly with the issues that arise from having so many limitations."

Some CFS patients seek out group therapy. In San Francisco, one such group meets at Operation Concern, headquartered in storefront offices on bustling Market Street, which provides mental health services to the city's highly visible lesbian and gay men's communities. The weekly meeting is targeted specifically at people with chronic illnesses and other disabilities and is attended by substantial numbers of CFS patients. Therapist Ricki Boden, who is visually impaired herself, talks about her special brand of group therapy:

> We provide a disabled assumption in a world in which there is an able-bodied assumption. For example, there is always the presumption of limitations, an acceptance that people will have better and worse days. You'll hear someone say, "Oh, your memory is not focused today. Let me repeat myself." Whether we are talking about relationships, work, or pursuing an education, everyone understands that health is always a factor in making a decision.

According to Boden, this therapeutic environment creates a basis from which patients can then learn to ask for accommodation in the larger world.

Survival Tactics

Whether you lean on a support group, turn to professional counseling, or rely on your own internal resources for strength, preserving your dignity and a sense of self-worth are crucial to your ability to cope. The advice that follows, supplied mostly from patients themselves, has that aim in mind.

Believe in Yourself

Rare is the CFS patient who in a moment of despair has not whispered, "Could my illness really reflect nothing more than stress or depression?" And in the space between moments of doubt, the specter of denial sometimes rears its ugly head. As one New Yorker explained:

> I never wanted to admit, even to myself, that I had a chronic illness. Its episodic pattern made it easier to deny the problem. I'd be sick for a couple of months, then well for six to eight weeks—and during each spate of good health, I'd convince myself that it could never happen again.

The symptoms of chronic fatigue syndrome can be so bizarre and the roller-coaster ride through illness and relative good health so erratic that it strains even your own credibility. But if you are to persuade others to believe in you—be they friends, family, doctors, or the administrators of the Social Security disability program—you must first believe in yourself. Do so by educating yourself about your illness and seeking out other patients who understand its peculiarities. Don't allow doubt to cloud your own vision. Remember that no one knows your body as well as you do and accept the signals it is sending.

Ask for Help

A passion for independence and a reluctance to ask for help are peculiar points of pride embedded deep within the American culture. "I was always Mr. Independent," said Peter B., a CFS patient. "It drove me crazy to have to ask for help. But then I felt irritated when others didn't sense my need and respond to it."

A craving for help and a reluctance to ask for it probably sounds familiar. To many CFS patients, it is a scenario sure to ring bells. Admitting weakness can be tough, but when life's most basic tasks— cooking, cleaning, and shopping, to say nothing of earning a living or caring for a family—become impossible there's not much choice but to learn how to request assistance.

Once you let go of your superachiever self-image and learn to admit "I can't," you may discover that reaching out to friends and family, articulating fear, and asking for practical and emotional support are signs of strength, not weakness. By acknowledging your interdependence and admitting need you open yourself to others and allow them to express their love for you. Many patients say it took a serious illness for them to realize just how crucial a personal support network is to their psychic survival.

Take the initiative in asking for help. Remember that despite their best intentions, your friends and family may not know just what to do for you or may fear that their efforts will be viewed as undue interference. Because CFS patients often do not look seriously ill, there is just no way that even your closest allies can realize how the simplest tasks sap you of energy—until you tell them so. There's more on the topic of close relationships and how to get what you need from them in the next chapter.

Admit Limitations

Sometimes CFS patients try to gloss over their symptoms and refuse to tell anyone just how badly they are really feeling. "I was always minimizing my problems," says one woman.

> I'd try to have dinner on the table the way I always had, even though exhaustion took a terrible toll as a result. Finally, I got to the point

where I said, "Enough of this. I have got to take care of *me* right now."
After that, I became much more vocal about drawing lines and talking
candidly about what I could and could not do.

Some CFS patients are guilty of wallowing in self-pity and they
are not very pleasant to be around. But if you are like the majority,
you'll err in a very different direction by trying to ignore your illness
and making unreasonable demands on yourself. For the sake of both
your emotional and physical health, pamper yourself a bit instead.
Concentrate your energies on what you do best and enjoy the most. It
is important to your sense of personal worth that you earn recognition
from others and take what pleasures you can at this difficult time in
your life.

Above all, don't make comparisons to your achievements when
you were in the prime of health. "I've finally stopped competing with
the late, great me," says one woman.

I just can't do what I used to do and there's no point in becoming
frustrated or cranky about it. I've learned to accept it and go on from
there. I do set goals but they are realistic goals that I can attain. I'll vow
to wash just one dish or telephone one old friend during the evening
and I'll get a real sense of achievement by accomplishing that aim.

Keep Laughing

Laughter has been called the music of life and it clearly helps release
some of the tension that accumulates with the daily struggle to cope
with chronic fatigue syndrome. As scientists develop a more sophisticated
understanding of the mind–body connection and the curative powers of
positive thinking, they are also coming to understand the physiological
basis for the benefits of laughter: a good belly laugh increases respiratory
activity, oxygen exchange, and heartbeat rate and may enhance the
system's ability to fight inflammation. Like exercise, it is also thought
to stimulate the brain to produce endorphins, a morphine-like chemical
that can increase one's sense of well-being and reduce depression.

Norman Cousins, editor of the *Saturday Review* for many years,
became a vocal advocate of laughter's curative powers after he was
diagnosed with a degenerative disease of the body's connective tissue.
In *Anatomy of an Illness,* he describes his decision to swear off traditional medications in favor of a treatment regimen of vitamin C and
belly laughter.

Cousin writes:

I made the joyous discovery that ten minutes of genuine belly laughter had an anesthetic effect and would give me at least two hours of pain-free sleep . . . Exactly what happens inside the human mind and body as the result of humor is difficult to say. But the evidence that it works has stimulated the speculations not just of physicians but of philosophers and scholars over the centuries.

According to Cousins, a belief in the powers of laughter dates back to the *Bible,* which says that a merry heart works like a doctor. Cousins also cites Immanuel Kant's claim that an individual who laughs heartily cannot become constipated and notes that a man as stern as Sigmund Freud believed that humor was an important therapeutic tool.

If laughter is indeed the best medicine, it is far better to chuckle than to cry over the peculiar memory lapses and momentary confusion that often characterize chronic fatigue syndrome. It's tough but it is also wise not to take yourself too seriously. Be frivolous, urges one man, a natural storyteller who entertains his support group with detailed descriptions of *Love Boat.* A favored cartoon, developed by a patient in Kansas City, shows what happens after a husband asks his wife to let the cat out and refrigerate the milk: A cat tail dangles out the refrigerator door and spoiled milk sits unnoticed on the porch.

Maintain a Sense of Purpose

With chronic illness comes a loss of identity and sometimes a loss of purpose. Maintaining a semblance of normal life—even if it just means attending one class a week or working an hour a day—is an important way of combating a sense of estrangement from the world around you. Patients who disengage entirely often become depressed and find it more difficult to return to normal activities as they recover.

Serving others in need is also rewarding. Until she learned to target her anger productively Janet Bohanon of Kansas City admits that it almost overwhelmed her: "You've got to learn to target all your pent-up emotions and fears and tears to help in a constructive way. Those of us who are ill are not lazy people. Many of us have been type A personalities and are used to always being active." Still she is not immune to the frustrations that inevitably accompany sickness. "There are so many things that I want to do, that my mind thinks it is capable of doing but the body won't go along with. It does depress me that I can't do what I really want," admits Bohanon.

Whether or not a cure is ever found for the illness that has plagued her and five members of her family for more than a decade, Janet Bohanon feels that CFS has radically altered her outlook: "I had gotten to the point where making money was the biggest thing in my life. My home was luxurious and my clothes were tailor-made but I had lost sight of the fact that we were put here to be our brother's keeper." She claims her leadership role in national and local support organizations had given her life new meaning by reminding her that "no matter how sick we are, we can all help someone."

Easy Does It

Coping effectively with chronic illness means changing your priorities and adjusting your lifestyle. "Both figuratively and literally, we can make a determined effort to refuse to be pushed by a crowd," says a social worker who counsels chronically ill patients. Working your way clear to emotional equilibrium means remaining calm in agitating situations, shrugging off the doubts of others, and gaining control over the tempo of your life. All easier said than done, of course, but for many it comes down to learning to relax and letting go of fears for the future.

In the throes of illness, worrying about your finances, your career, or your prospects for marriage only wastes precious energy. For now, let the accomplishments of the moment be sufficient and allow the disappointments to pass without undue concern. Hold tight to the knowledge that you are likely to recover from chronic fatigue syndrome and then there will be time enough to plan for the future. Keep your eye on the donut, not on the hole. "There are moments when I feel pessimistic, everything seems very black but I hold on until it passes and then I get very optimistic again," says New Yorker Condy Eckerle. "I think that because of all this, I'll emerge with a deeper understanding of what it means to be successful and happy in life."

The Challenge of Recovery

Although CFS patients wait, hope, and work for it, recovery, when it comes, poses its own challenges. Getting back into the swing of things after an involuntary absence, particularly one of several years duration, is not easy. Sara L., a Detroit woman who was forced to leave her teaching post and live off a small inheritance says:

I feel as though I have lost my center of gravity from being out of commission for so long. My self-identify is a little adrift. It's hard to know how to reestablish ties with the real world. Not working has become stressful now, but I know I need to be careful about jumping into something full blast. I don't want to endure a backlash in reaction.

Since physical recovery usually comes in incremental stages, you may still need some special consideration at work or on the social circuit. How do you explain a prolonged illness to a potential employer? What do you say about your recent bout of sickness to that special someone who catches your eye? What happens to the dynamics of a relationship that has been based on dependence and need, rather than on strength and good health?

We can provide no ready answers, only suggest that the questions merit careful consideration. Because post-CFS adjustment can be so challenging, some patients opt for psychological counseling *after* the worst of the illness has passed. That's when Nick R. chose to see a therapist:

I was convinced that my illness had an organic basis and I didn't feel that therapy could help me through it. But as I began to recover, therapy took on a new value as a means of building my self-esteem back up. I've got a lot of anxiety about what kind of work I'll be able to peg into and it really helps to be able to talk about that.

Others find the emotional sustenance to ease back into the world from the same friends and family who stood by during the long course of the illness. "A few kind words really helped get me through," said Liz B. "I needed to hear that there would be an end to this thing and my family was always there to tell me so." In the next chapter, we'll talk more about how personal relationships are affected by chronic fatigue syndrome and take a closer look at ways you can get the help you need from those you love.

7

∎

A Helping Hand:
Getting What You Need from
Friends and Family

You don't just have this illness alone. Your whole family has it. It changes everyone's life.

–Terry G., CFS patient,
Terre Haute, Indiana

I desperately wanted people to believe me when I talked about how I had been ravaged by chronic fatigue syndrome. I also pleaded with them to understand that the illness was not something I could control. But what I wanted most of all was candor—I wanted my friends to tell me how they felt about CFS and how it was affecting our relationships. The subject seemed to make people nervous, though— they'd try to change the topic as though they could pretend it wasn't really happening.

–Rhoda S., CFS patient,
Los Angeles, California

Those who have weathered the debilitating effects of chronic fatigue syndrome most often heap credit on their loved ones. Toni D., a thirty-eight-year-old businesswoman from Chicago, considers herself lucky. Until falling ill at the age of thirty-eight, she ran a small export–import firm and juggled the tasks of maintaining a four-person household as well. Although she has continued to work, albeit on a much reduced schedule, CFS forced her to curtail many other activities. "I'd never have pulled through without Ted," says Toni, calling her husband's support crucial to her emotional well-being. "When I couldn't handle something, he'd handle it for me. He really viewed our marriage as teamwork and his faith in my recovery helped sustain me."

Many chronic fatigue syndrome patients are not as lucky. The illness is notorious for placing a strain on personal relationships. The annals of CFS history are rife with stories about friends and family members who express incessant skepticism about the condition, lose patience as the symptoms drag on over months and years, or withdraw emotionally. Tales of shattered love, familial estrangement, and broken friendships are told with alarming frequency.

Asking for—and getting—the help that you need from others is one of the greatest challenges of chronic illness. It is not mere happenstance that certain marriages and some friendships last while others are torn apart as CFS runs its course. The ones that endure are those in which all parties remain sensitive to their own emotions, admitting anger and fear as each arises, and struggling over sensitive issues, rather than evading them. The couples who reach common ground, the parents and children who achieve heightened levels of understanding, and the friends who cast their bonds of loyalty in stone are those who manage—in good times and bad—to keep open the lines of communication between them.

How CFS Affects Close Relationships

It is far easier for friends and family to behave heroically during a short-term crisis than to muster the emotional energy necessary to provide support over the long haul of a chronic illness. In an emergency, pressing and well-defined needs must usually be met quickly; once a crisis is resolved, life continues much as in the past. Coping with a long-term illness is very different. By definition open-ended, it is impossible to say just when—if ever—life will be as it was in the golden days of good health.

The peculiarities of CFS present more than even the usual challenges. Patients are likely to feel estranged and misunderstood. "No one who is healthy can understand what it's like to be sick every day," complained one man, encapsulating the cause of so much alienation between the well and the ill. Although we'd like to believe that our loved ones have utmost faith in us, a certain stigma still attaches to chronic fatigue syndrome because it has been so plagued by credibility problems. Whether or not they stand by your side, your spouse, your close friends, and even your parents may silently harbor doubts as to just how real your complaints are—or you may wonder if they do. The possibility that chronic fatigue syndrome is contagious provokes an equally irrational response. The opinions of medical experts—who doubt CFS can be casually transmitted—do little to reduce fear. "You waste energy trying to convince others that you're really sick and once they finally believe you, they may not want to have anything to do with you," said a disgruntled teenage patient. In a society where people have spoken openly about tattooing AIDS patients, the nagging questions that linger about contagion leave patients feeling tainted and vulnerable.

The Taint of Sickness

In our individualistic society, with its emphasis on youth and good health, there is generally an enormous reluctance to deal with illness. Healthy people often prefer to bury their heads in the sands of denial rather than to face the haunting specter of disease and the thoughts of mortality that it fuels. One San Francisco man says that in his heyday of good health, he was known as a social butterfly, at the center of a wide circle of friends. After he fell ill, an overactive gossip mill spread wild rumors—one day word was out that Randy P. had AIDS. Next it was said that he had a brain tumor. Some people heard that he died. Incredibly, most of his friends were afraid to call to express concern or to get the story straight.

"A lot of people just don't want to hear about illness. They aren't prepared to deal with it. Or they will believe you are crazy. Or they will believe it is AIDS no matter what you tell them," said CFS patient Janet K. Rather than admitting that fate is fickle and anyone is vulnerable to disease—both highly threatening notions—it is human nature to believe that sickness only happens to someone else. As a result, we become suspicious of sick people themselves, as if their misfortune was entirely self-inflicted. "People have an odd attitude toward illness," said patient leader Bob Landau. "They somehow believe that you want to be sick. It is part of the unfortunate fiction that most of us subscribe to that we can control our lives."

Just as adulterers were onced forced to wear the scarlet letter "A," so CFS patients seem marked with a "D," symbolizing the fact that they are diseased. Thus stigmatized, it is little wonder that personal connections often become bent out of shape, and sometimes broken.

Why Close Bonds Are Strained

It often comes as a shock to discover how deeply your friends and family are affected by your misfortune and how much they grieve. "It tears me up to watch my son have to deal with this," said one gentleman, who was attending a CFS support group meeting because his twenty-two-year-old son was too ill to come. Alas, empathetic grief is rarely all that your loved ones feel. No matter how irrational or unfair, frustration and rage often vie with compassion for control over their emotional state.

Family dynamics suffer the greatest dislocations when one partner is felled by CFS. Agreed-upon divisions of responsibilities within a family may no longer be viable and new agreements will have to be inked. Young children are likely to feel bewildered and threatened and will need special attention and reassurance. Just when you most need a stable and loving partner, your spouse may become distant and resentful. Hopes and dreams for the future, a natural part of any marriage, often come crashing down in the wake of chronic fatigue syndrome. At the same time, a waning interest in sex is likely to drive a further wedge between you.

In the previous chapter we talked about how the syndrome inflicts grievous wounds on your self-image. Whether you have been a breadwinner or a homemaker, CFS also shatters the vision others have had of you. You may have to ask family members to do things that you once did easily for yourself; that means they will have to restructure their own lives in order to fill your shoes. And you may be unable to devote your full energies to your children, who rely on you for both practical and emotional support; as a result, they may feel let down or shunted aside.

Friendships that have been based principally on casual socializing may weaken when you are unable to share hobbies, sports, or shopping. "We can be depressing to someone who is well," admits one patient, pointing out that most young, healthy people haven't had much firsthand experience with serious illness and often don't know how to cope with it. "There's not really any retort I can make when my friends groan at my complaints and say 'you're just no fun any more.' " Your friends may also be nervous and unsure of themselves in your presence, not knowing exactly what to say or how to help.

The fact that the illness isn't readily apparent to a casual observer can be more a curse than a blessing. Many patients have come to detest the well-meaning phrase "you look great" because it implies, "you can't really be feeling too badly." Vague doubts about the legitimacy of the syndrome also surface when patients are unable to make firm plans or honor their commitments. The real reason why—because the unpredictability of the symptoms lays determination and good intentions to waste—sometimes gets lost in a wave of resentment and suspicion. Friends and family may secretly suspect you are using illness as an excuse to avoid doing something you don't really want to do, and that is certain to add fuel to the fires of tension.

One ailing woman describes the straw that broke the back of her ten-year marriage.

> Things really turned sour for us after I canceled out on his brother's wedding. I know how badly he wanted me to go and I rested up well ahead of time. But my legs were like jelly that day and I felt so dizzy I thought I'd topple over. It just wasn't possible for me to make it and I don't think he ever forgave me.

Perhaps most stressful to any relationship is the fact that no one can predict how long these accumulated pressures will last. A year? Five years? Ten years? Or forever? Given the uncertain course of CFS, no one can realistically say.

When Friends and Family Don't Come Through

When those you love turn cold or indifferent, the ensuing pain can be searing. Patients express disappointment and sometimes rage toward friends who don't come through. Phyllis S., age forty-one, talked about friends she had known for twenty years who failed her when the chips were down. "Lots of people think this whole thing is a figment of my imagination. They accuse me of making too much out of it." Her voice shook with anger as she demanded, "How dare someone question the legitimacy of how I feel? Out of loyalty alone these people should believe me. Since I fell ill, a great many people have managed to alienate themselves from me."

Through their experiences with CFS, many people learn the painful truth that when we laugh, the world will usually laugh with us, but when we cry, we often cry alone. "Many people do lose a lot of connections with friends and family if they condition those relationships on their response to illness," says San Francisco social worker Ricki Boden. "Other people are able to continue certain relationships only because they accept their limitations."

While healthy friends and family should provide crucial strength and support to you—and you have every right to be disappointed if they fail to do so—there is much emotional healing and psychic rebuilding that can only be done by turning inward for strength. Don't ask more than is reasonable from those you love: No matter how close the relationship, no one can travel with you along the whole jagged journey toward good health. Ultimately you must walk part of the distance alone.

Keeping Close Ties

Although a bout with chronic fatigue syndrome might seem a high price to pay for a lesson in human relations, many patients say their experiences have given them new insights into the role of intimacy, candor, and trust in interpersonal relationships. "I'm more willing to give people the benefit of the doubt on any score now," said Nick R., a Queens, New York man who credits homeopathy for his radical improvement in health. Nick believes his struggle with the ravages of CFS has deepened his compassion for others. "Having been subjected to the idea that this thing could all be psychological, I'm a lot more inclined now to listen and to really respect what others are telling me."

Here are some ways to make the best out of your painful struggles with chronic illness and to emerge with most of your relationships intact, perhaps even strengthened.

The Whole Truth and Nothing But

Frank, not histrionic, communication is the single most effective way to get what you need from your friends and family. Some people fear they will drive away those who are closest to them by talking too much about illness, especially because the symptoms are so vague and the prognosis is so uncertain. In fact, the opposite is probably true: Not knowing what is wrong or how to help frightens and isolates people who love you. Keep others informed about your health problems. Asking explicitly for what you need makes it much more likely that you'll get it. "In the first year that I was ill, I did a lot of damage to my closest relationships," admitted one man. "It seemed to me that my friends weren't responding well to my needs and I was resentful and hostile in return. It was a long time before I realized that I was forcing them to guess what I needed."

Obviously there are a lot of questions to which the answers are unknown. You can't predict the full course of your illness or speculate on just what changes it will bring to your life. But you can explain current medical thinking, talk about the treatments that are being recommended for you, and discuss other patient experiences you have heard about. Having candid conversations with confidants is also a useful way for you to get in touch with your own feelings and fears.

Steer Away from the Guilt Trip

The ugly specter of guilt is often raised during the course of a chronic illness. As a patient, it is common to suffer guilt pangs because you feel yourself a burden to others, constantly asking for help, and frequently unable to hold up your end of a relationship bargain. At the same time, you may resent that situation and your resentment can flare into accusations like, "You don't pay enough attention to me" or, "You get to have all the fun."

Often it is difficult to know how candid to be when asked about your health. "If I tell my husband how I really feel, I feel guilty for putting that burden on him," said one peppy woman who has been ill for more than a year. "On the other hand, I don't think it is fair to have to hide my condition from someone I love. Sometimes I just feel that if he can't deal with the truth, I'll find someone who can."

Those who love you also struggle with feelings of guilt—no matter how much they do, it may not be enough to meet all your needs. If they go out after work or attend a party alone, they may feel they have been disloyal to you. The pressure of trying to provide the help you need, coupled with the other stresses of daily life, may cause your partner to snap at you in irritation—and immediately afterward, to feel guilty about having done so.

Guilt is highly counterproductive and virtually guaranteed to distort the dynamics of any relationship, but it does its greatest damage to a marriage. It is not your fault that you are ill, nor is it in your partner's power to wave away the symptoms with a magic wand. As long as either one of you suffers pangs of contrition or wastes time looking for scapegoats, you won't have energy left over to make the long-term adjustments that chronic fatigue syndrome demands.

Appropriate Behavior:
Yours and Theirs

It is not easy for friends and family to watch you suffer or cope with limitations. Have some compassion for their pain and remember that your own moods cast a shadow on the lives of those around you. While you don't need to stifle your own fear and grief, it is important to channel your frustrations so that you don't lash out irrationally at those around you.

On the other hand, don't let those you love off the hook too readily. A tremendous amount of resentment can build up when people respond inappropriately to your illness. Although confrontation may strain your limited energy, letting an uncomfortable situation eat away at you ultimately creates even more stress—and that's unhealthy for everyone. If tensions are driving a wedge between you and someone that you love, don't hesitate to call in an objective outsider—a counselor, minister, or just a friend—to serve as mediator in ironing out some of the tensions that arise.

"My wife is a nurse but I felt as if she was using up all her compassion on her patients," said Paul B., whose marriage was poised on the edge of disintegration as his CFS symptoms dragged into their fourth year. "At first she tried to be supportive but gradually I could feel her drawing back from me. We were stultifyingly polite to each other but we weren't communicating." Fortunately, Paul and his wife sought counseling from a therapist with a special interest in physical disabilities and were able to peel back the layers of unspoken hostility and deal effectively with some of the issues causing them both such consternation.

Remember That Your Spouse
Has Needs

Sometimes an ailing person becomes so dependent on a spouse that the healthy partner's needs get neglected. It is easy to understand why: When the simplest routines involve enormous struggle and your drive to get well assumes primary importance in your life, it is hard not to become self-involved. In the long run, though, focusing single-mindedly on your own health can destroy other relationships.

No matter how needy you feel, remember that your husband, wife, or lover deserves some respect and attention, too. Encourage your loved ones in their own pursuits and remind them that what they are doing is of importance and interest to you. Ask about their activities outside the home. "I'm disabled but I can still make a contribution," says one patient. "My lover may be doing my laundry for me but I'm there to congratulate him when good things happen and to commiserate with his disappointments. Physically I can't do much but emotionally I still try to offer a lot."

No matter how dedicated, every care-giver needs occasional time off. Taking vacations alone has become commonplace for the spouses of many CFS patients. Encouraging your mate to get away for a weekend or a week at a time—preferably *before* the need for a break becomes too desperate—is a good way to provide you both a respite and to prevent a lover from feeling too put-upon. "I have to have a week by myself," one frazzled husband told his ailing wife. "A week where I don't have to worry about you, about the business, about anything at all." The healing power of his week alone proved so refreshing that he returned home with the energy to shoulder his double-duty responsibilities again.

The Delicate Sexual Arena

On top of all the other strains that chronic fatigue syndrome places on a relationship, many people find they lack both energy and interest in sex. Intercourse is physically demanding, and like other strenuous activities, it often extracts a toll in exhaustion that costs CFS patients dearly for several days afterward. But the loss of physical intimacy at a time when a partner already resents the burdens of care-giving can have devastating consequences.

Raise the issue of sex before unspoken tensions about it erupt into an ugly scene. Talk candidly about the problem, the limitations on your energy, and your alternatives. Let your partner know how much gentle physical affection means to you: Touching, hugging, and kissing are soothing reminders of your self-worth and reassurance that you are still desirable. Be imaginative in your approach to sex. Oral and manual stimulation are often a less tiring form of lovemaking and increasing luxuriant foreplay and tenderness may allow you to shorten the more enervating sexual intercourse without either partner feeling slighted. Certain positions enable the ill partner to be more passive and relaxed while still giving pleasure. You may also want to try making love when your energy level is at its peak, rather than pigeonholing sex as a nighttime activity, when even healthy people feel weary.

What to Tell the Children

Unless the issues that arise are handled properly, your children can be as victimized by chronic illness as you are. Unerringly perceptive, they have a knack for sensing when something is wrong, even if they are not necessarily mature enough to understand just what it is. Efforts to hide illness from children usually backfire, stimulating nightmarish fantasies or making them believe they are to blame for the changed household mood.

Avoid these problems by talking candidly with your children about chronic fatigue syndrome, using concepts and analogies they can understand. Because your changing symptoms will affect the family dynamics differently at different times, communication is an ongoing process. Your children are likely to pepper you with unanswerable questions: How long will you be sick? What caused the sickness? Will I get sick, too? Be as truthful as possible without fueling further fears. Indicate that most people do recover from CFS, although it may take a long while, and let them know that scientists are working hard to learn more about the cause and cure. Given all the medical uncertainties, there's no reason whatsoever to tell healthy children that CFS sometimes runs in families.

During the course of your illness, keep a close eye for how your children are coping: Acting out, severe changes in eating or sleeping patterns, and difficulty in school all suggest they are feeling unduly threatened by your illness and need special attention.

Who Will Love Me Now?

One chronic fatigue syndrome patient in her early thirties, a hard-driven career woman who had deliberately postponed marriage and childbearing while she pursued professional goals, spoke for a host of victims when she cried, "Who will love me now?"

As intensely as CFS strains the commitment of a marriage or a long-term relationship, some think it extracts an even harsher toll on single men and women. Meeting new people becomes almost impossible when most of your energies are consumed by the day-to-day struggle for survival. Confidence and a positive self-image are in short supply when you are in the throes of a battle against chronic fatigue syndrome, which makes it difficult to pursue someone who does catch your eye.

In the age of AIDS, connecting with strangers has taken on a heightened risk. The odds that a budding romance will wither once your would-be amour realizes the severity of your illness has increased. Fear that you are contaminated by disease is a major concern— subconsciously, you may half believe it yourself, a fear you can't help projecting to others. Many patients can relate to the story told by Tom P. at one support group meeting: "I decided to be candid about chronic fatigue syndrome and the limitations it imposed on me. But when I explained it to a woman I was really interested in, she said 'well, that certainly sounds contagious' and turned me down for future dates."

This situation raises a particularly irksome issue: When should you tell a potential lover about the syndrome? Robert P., who walks slowly and tentatively in order to control his dizziness, usually excuses himself by telling a first date that he has a bad back. But he feels badly about the deceit. "I'm used to being honest and here I am lying to her at the very beginning of a potential relationship," says Robert.

Faced with these compound problems, some people hesitate to turn down even the most unsuitable candidate for a relationship, fearing the chance might not come again. "Sometimes I ask myself, 'Who am I to be so picky right now?' " says one man. Rather than risk rejection or loneliness people find themselves lingering in relationships that have run their course or making commitments for all the wrong reasons. "I've gotten involved in a new relationship but I'm not at all sure that it is the right one for me," says one thirty-eight-year-old woman. "I've become very dependent on Jerry because he is a genuinely nice guy and he's helpful but I don't think we'd be together under other circumstances. Still the thought of being alone and having to cope by myself is very unappealing."

Although the temptation to compromise is understandable, settling for a relationship that is not all you need or want is doomed to failure. A relationship built on dependency often doesn't last once you begin to recover your health. Having become accustomed to a role as a caretaker, it is difficult for your partner to adjust to your hard-won independence. The only way to develop the successful relationship that will sustain you in sickness *and* in health is to trust your intuition, apply the same standards you would if you were healthy, and above all, communicate, communicate, communicate!

Moving Back with Your Parents

Unable to cope emotionally or financially, some patients return to the homes of their parents to recuperate. Patient leader Bob Landau, who had worked his way through college and always prided himself on his financial independence, decided to move back in with his mother when he became virtually bedridden. Although he was reluctant to give up his apartment, the precarious state of his health simply left him no alternative. Nonetheless, Landau opted to pay rent from his work-related disability insurance. "It was very important to me that I pay my own way as much as I could. It was enough that I was being an emotional stress to my mother, I didn't want to put her in the poorhouse as well."

After years of independence, the decision to return to mom and dad is not an easy one to make. Landau says, "Parents tend to be forced back into being parents again. They can't help but be the caretakers of their children. And it forces those of us who are trying to be adults into being helpless children instead. It's like being on an allowance again."

When moving back with the folks is the best alternative you've got, there are some steps you can take to see that the arrangement will work smoothly:

- Talk candidly about your health situation and your reasons for moving back home. Now, more than ever, you need emotional support and encouragement from your parents. Be certain that they understand the latest medical thinking about chronic fatigue syndrome and appreciate how difficult it is to predict recovery.

- Clarify the financial and work arrangements within the household. If you are able to make a financial contribution to the running expenses of the house, it may help to eliminate any tension on this issue. Try to help out in any way you can. If cooking and cleaning are impossible, folding the laundry, repairing a broken dish, or doing some sewing would be equally appreciated.

- Agree on household rules. If you've lived away from home for any length of time, it will not be easy to accept restrictions on your lifestyle. But there are likely to be times when you feel well enough to go out for the evening—or perhaps would like a guest to stay overnight. A candid discussion about curfews and visitors will stave off future tension on these subjects.

An Aside to Those Who Love CFS Patients*

If chronic fatigue syndrome is a witch's brew of misery, a patient sometimes feels like a bundle of needs. One man spoke the desperation of thousands when he said, "We need far more help than our families can possibly be expected to give us."

Maybe so, but if you love someone who has CFS, there are numerous concrete things you can do. Assisting with basic household tasks and providing the assertive companionship necessary to maneuver through the maze of medical bureaucracy can be invaluable. Remember how difficult it is to say "I can't!" and "please help"; shoulder extra responsibilities *before* being asked to do so. Understand your loved one's limitations and make it a point to praise accomplishments rather than belittle failure. When necessary, provide a sympathetic ear and a shoulder to cry on.

Here is a detailed look at other ways to ease a patient's journey safely past the shoals of illness—and strengthen the ties holding you together at the same time.

Learn as much as possible about CFS. New information about the cause and proper treatment of chronic fatigue syndrome is being uncovered every day. Subscribing to one of the national association newsletters is a good way to stay informed about current medical findings and to let the patient know you acknowledge the illness and care about what's being done to cure it. Ignorance breeds fear and you can also relieve some of your own concerns—about the prospects for recovery and the likelihood of contagion, for examples—by getting the real facts.

Communicate openly. Some friends and relatives deal with CFS by ignoring it. It's fine to be cheerful and optimistic but don't bury your head in the sand of denial. CFS patients need to talk about their physical and psychic well-being and usually appreciate your tactful questions and genuine efforts to understand their feelings. Don't get nervous when the topic arises and don't try to change the subject at the earliest opportunity.

Get involved in the work of your local support group. Most groups are in desperate need of able-bodied volunteers to help set up meetings, arrange for speakers, organize letter-writing campaigns, and respond

*Psst! CFS patients: You may want to show this section to someone you love.

to requests for information from patients, the media, and others. Orvalene Prewitt, who heads the National CFS Association in Kansas City, first became involved in chronic fatigue syndrome support work because her husband was ill. "This illness took so much away from us," she says with regret. "By getting involved in trying to find some answers, you are doing something to really fight the illness, you have some kind of control over it. After all, it is my family that is at stake here."

Don't be condescending or bossy. Because someone is physically sick doesn't mean that he or she has the intellectual capacity of a two-year-old. Remember, CFS patients have lost a great deal of independence already and do not need to have their last shred of dignity and autonomy challenged. Advice is fine; dictatorial demands are not.

Help keep patients in touch with the outside world. Like the elderly, chronically ill people who lose much of their mobility tend to become insular and self-involved. They may lose touch with news of their community, trends in fashion, art, and cuisine, or political developments. By providing appropriate reading material or telling tales about the world beyond the boundaries of their home, you can keep patients up to date on changing trends and help reduce their isolation.

Accept the limitations imposed by CFS. Whatever else it may be, the syndrome is unpredictable. Your loved one may rest up for two days in preparation for an important event—and still not feel up to going. Or a person may have to rest so frequently while doing household chores that projects go unfinished. Try not to lost patience, remembering how much more frustrating the situation is for the ailing person. It's okay to feel disappointment but launching a tirade of anger or laying blame just isn't fair. It is not as though your mate can do much to change the situation. Remember also that the line between gentle prodding and nagging is a blurry one and don't fuel resentment by suggesting that hard work or an optimistic attitude are all that is needed for recovery.

Be flexible. As the late John Lennon told us long ago, life is what happens to you when you are busy making other plans. CFS changes the lives of everyone it touches no matter how carefully those lives have been arranged. The sooner you come to grips with this reality, the better off all concerned parties will be. An ailing wife accustomed to doing all the housework may suddenly depend on her husband to cook and clean. The chores of household maintenance that traditionally fell to a husband may have to be delegated to others. Adjustment doesn't come easily and you can't cope if you're not flexible.

Remember, CFS patients need breathing room, too. No matter how well-intentioned, don't suffocate the person you love. Less catastrophic than neglect, it is nonetheless imperative to remember that sick people don't always have the energy to deal with others around them. Visit, help out, and bring good cheer, but don't wear out the patient—and your own welcome.

Insist on time for yourself. Burnout is a major problem among care-givers, who often run themselves ragged trying to do the work of two people. Although your devotion is undoubtedly well-intended and thoroughly appreciated, it can become counterproductive. Chances are that you'll ultimately reach a breaking point where you're unable to continue. Before you exceed the limits of your energy, talk with your loved one about when and how your help is needed. Be sure to schedule regular time off. Try to get other friends or family members to share the caretaking role. Spreading the burden not only relieves you of full responsibility, it also gives others a chance to show how much they care.

[   ]

Chronic fatigue syndrome makes enormous demands on anyone it touches, but there is no overestimating the importance of outside help. "There is a line of demarcation between patients who have a supportive family and those who do not. Those who do cope so much better," emphasizes Marc Iverson, who heads the Chronic Fatigue and Immune Dysfunction Syndrome (CFIDS) Association in Charlotte, North Carolina. "It is so moving when I hear about a parent or a spouse who says 'I'll be with you all the way.' "

Emotional sustenance and strong social connections are key elements in the package of patient needs. Financial realities are also a major concern. The way in which CFS patients function on the job and how they manage financially if working becomes impossible can make a crucial difference to the speed of recovery.

8

■

Coping with Work
and What to Do When
You Can't: A Guide to
Financial Survival

It almost killed me when I was forced to go on a leave of absence. I had finally reached a point in my career that I had been working for all my life. And I felt like I was a parasite. I had always been a productive member of society and now I was nothing.

–Mimi Tipton, CFS support group leader,
Newark, Delaware

One of the greatest indignities of our health care system is that we feel compelled to continue working in order to hold on to our health insurance at the same time that we are coping with an overpowering illness.

–Geoff R., CFS patient,
San Francisco, California

Along with the physical and psychic discomfort of chronic fatigue syndrome, patients very often face tremendous financial hardships. Many victims of this perplexing syndrome have been financially secure all their lives and are unprepared for the economic dislocation that is often the consequence of an extended disability. Soaring health care expenses and plummeting earnings capacity mean a mountain of bills and no revenue with which to pay them.

Patients who find it impossible to hold down a job once they become ill may face dire financial consequences. Dwindling assets and the loss of employment-linked health insurance quickly pose a plethora of never-before asked questions: What am I going to do about all my bills? How can I pay for reputable health care? What are personal bankruptcy proceedings all about? Will I ever be employable again?

There are no easy answers to any of these questions but fortunately there are a number of federal, state, and local benefits available for people in need. Although the heart of the American safety net has been weakened in recent years, Social Security disability payments, Medicare, Medicaid, and various social welfare programs still provide some income and health care guarantees. Chronic fatigue syndrome patients also qualify for many of the services and legal protections available to other disabled persons. In this chapter, we'll look first at the challenge of remaining in the workplace while enduring the unpredictable fluctuations of chronic fatigue syndrome, and then discuss financial strategies for staying afloat without an income.

Coping in the Workplace

The career-oriented professionals who seem to be at highest risk for CFS have earned their positions by virtue of talent, commitment, and hard work and the prospect of losing it all can be devastating. But staying in a physically or emotionally stressful job can also extract a brutal toll in the form of exacerbated symptoms and lengthened recuperation time.

When it is medically feasible, the advantages of continuing to work are obvious: A good job enhances your sense of personal value, distracts you from the self-absorption that often accompanies chronic illness, and provides greater financial security. But exceeding your limits or trying to cope in a pressure-cooker work environment without the armor of your full strength isn't worth the cost. Sandra B., a thirty-five-year-old Washington, D.C. woman, learned this lesson the hard way. An executive secretary for a wealthy philanthropist, she clung to her position long after it was medically sound to do so. Part of the reason was pride and a reluctance to admit that she was defeated by illness. Her boss's lack of compassion did not help matters any. The former secretary explains:

> My boss wasn't the least bit sympathetic or understanding. He said, "Well you look fine to me," so I pushed myself beyond my limits and went to work every single day. The bill has come due for that decision now. You really can't work when you are ill without paying serious consequences for it.

And yet quitting a job, abandoning an avocational passion, or dropping out of school means setting aside your aspirations and dreams, which also has a high price. "Art was my religion. It was a very spiritual connection for me. To lose that connectedness has been a very devastating experience," says a forty-five-year-old sculptor whose huge wooden pieces earned her a listing in *Contemporary American Women Sculptors*. Now even carrying a sketchbook has become too much of a physical strain and most of her days are spent in the isolation of a tiny, dark, studio apartment in Manhattan.

For some patients, of course, the employment question is moot. Once a powerhouse media executive, Belle H. now admits, "I would not employ me. You have to be well in the work world. Do you want to hire someone who has the flu every day? Or someone who has to lie on the sofa for three hours in the afternoon? Most of us have become unemployable."

If you do stay on the job, often struggling along at reduced capacity, you'll probably have to make some explanations to your co-workers. The AIDS bugaboo invariably rears its ugly head, with some CFS patients reporting that they have been ostracized by ignorant colleagues fearful of contagion. One employee spent an hour with his boss trying to describe the enigma of chronic fatigue syndrome and the ways in which it limited his job performance. Exasperated, his boss finally exploded, "Why couldn't you just have broken a leg?" The implication—that a broken bone is tangible and finite, easy to understand, and predictable in its course, while CFS is mysterious and somehow suspect—is something that patients have to cope with all the time.

For these and other reasons, many chronic fatigue syndrome patients try not to let their colleagues know how sick they are. But hiding the truth is far from ideal. Sometimes patients find themselves resented by co-workers who perceive them to be doing the barest minimum. Others pay the price in exhaustion. "I felt as if I were living a double life, pretending to be healthy at work, then coming home to collapse. I slept almost straight through every weekend and even then I had to drag myself into the office on Monday morning," said Sandi, age thirty-eight, an editor who quit her job after a year of illness when she could no longer sustain the charade of good health.

Arranging to work part-time is one solution to the workplace dilemma. A reduced work schedule can ease the problems of isolation and fear associated with chronic fatigue syndrome yet spare you the strain of a full-time job. It also smoothes the adjustment back to normalcy as you recover, and financially it is a lot easier than earning no paycheck at all, especially if you can negotiate for the continuation of your health benefits. Requesting a leave of absence is another way to keep your employment options open.

Convincing an employer to create a part-time position or to leave options available has not traditionally been an easy task, especially when the duration of the arrangement is open-ended. However, flexible scheduling arrangements have gained popularity in recent years, as thousands of working women seek new ways to fulfill career and family responsibilities. If your firm accommodates working mothers, they may also be flexible enough to extend the benefits of a reduced work schedule or a leave of absence to you.

If you are too disabled to work, you may qualify for corporate disability benefits on either a long-term or a short-term basis. Disability plans vary, of course, but with proper certification from your physician many companies will pay at least a portion of your salary, sometimes for a year or longer. Before leaving your job, be certain to discuss your right to disability with the company's benefit office or your union representative.

No Work, No Coverage:
The Health Insurance Trap

Almost alone among industrialized countries, the United States makes no provisions for national health insurance, forcing many chronic fatigue syndrome patients to confront one of the tragic ironies of our health care system: Individuals who are too ill to work stand to lose their insurance coverage at the very moment they need it most.

In 1986, the United States Congress took a small step toward changing the situation. Under the Comprehensive Budget Reconciliation Act (COBRA), an employee who leaves a job under almost any circumstances can continue to receive coverage through an employer's group health insurance plan for a period of eighteen months by assuming the cost of the premiums. While the new federal legislation falls far short of national health insurance, it does provide access, albeit on a temporary basis, to group health insurance, which almost always provides better coverage at lower rates than an individual policy.

If your job provides no health benefits or you have passed the eighteen-month cutoff, you may be able to purchase insurance at a group rate through a professional association. Writers' and artists' organizations, for example, often offer insurance plans, or you may be able to obtain coverage through a club, church group, or union. Most insurance companies, however, exclude payment for "preexisting conditions" so if you have already run up big medical bills for the diagnosis or treatment of chronic fatigue syndrome, finding an affordable plan becomes nearly impossible.

If you are lucky enough to be able to afford private health insurance, poor enough to qualify for Medicaid, or sick enough to be covered under Medicare (both programs are described later in this chapter), most of your bills for physician care, hospitalization, and medication will be covered. However, chronically ill people need a great many other health and social services that are not subsidized as readily. In order for CFS patients to have the long hours of stress-free rest that are a crucial part of building back strength, home health care, personal care services, and care-giver respite can be invaluable. If these services are unavailable or unaffordable, struggling with the logistics of daily living and the hassle of traveling to medical appointments almost certainly postpones recovery.

Until systemwide policy changes are made to improve access to affordable health care—and some CFS organizations are linking with other groups to help push for these changes—haunting concerns about access to appropriate care surface time and time again. For now, below is a review of some public benefits programs that can literally spell the difference between financial survival and calamity.

Public Benefits Programs

The decision to apply for public assistance does not come easily to CFS patients, who have typically been self-sufficient for many years. While you may initially balk at the prospect, it is an error to view government benefits as a handout. Your tax dollars have almost assuredly subsidized these benefits for others over the years and there is no shame in asking for your fair share when it becomes necessary.

A more real problem is how to cope with the formidable bureaucracy that stands guard over many public programs. The mechanisms for determining eligibility are complex and the hassles of applying for benefits, waiting on lines, and coping with interviews in which intimate details of your life are discussed is not a pleasant prospect, especially when you are already weakened by illness. Prepare yourself for the application process by reading about federal and state entitlement programs, and if possible, by talking to others who have gone through eligibility interviews. Try not to tackle the whole project alone. A friend or family member can certainly accompany you to a government office and may even be permitted to attend the interview and intercede on your behalf. Some patients sign over "power of attorney" to a trusted friend or relative, who can then represent them in all their legal dealings. And many of the support groups can provide a patient advocate to help you negotiate your way through the system.

Applying for Social Security Disability

Anyone deemed too incapacitated to perform even sedentary labor may be entitled to a monthly stipend under the provisions of the Social Security disability program. Eligibility standards are strict, however. According to the Social Security Administration (SSA):

> A person is considered disabled when he or she has a severe physical or mental impairment or combination of impairments that prevents him or her from working for a year or more or that is expected to result in death. The work does not necessarily have to be the kind of work done before disability—it can be any gainful work found in the national economy. This definition requires total disability.

Social Security disability benefits are funded through the Social Security taxes paid by employees, employers, and self-employed people. Thus, to be eligible for Social Security disability benefits, an individual must have worked long enough and recently enough to be insured under the system. A formula that factors in age, income level, and amount of time worked is used to determine preliminary eligibility so that individuals who don't qualify need not go through the rigors of the application process.

Although chronic fatigue syndrome was added to the Social Security Administration's list of officially recognized illnesses in 1988 (Section 24575.005, Chapter 245 of the *Program Operations Manual* under the name chronic Epstein-Barr virus syndrome), disability decisions for CFS patients remain inconsistent and unpredictable. Indeed criteria for granting disability benefits to CFS patients have been so murky that Congress recently called on the SSA to clean up its act, agree on a consistent definition of CFS, and promulgate better guidelines.

Two excellent sources of further information—*Social Security Disability Benefits: How to Get Them, How to Keep Them* by James Ross and

"Social Security Benefits and Chronic Fatigue Syndrome" by Samuel
Imperati and Janis Person—are listed in Appendix C.

Building a Case. Until SSA spells out its eligibility terms, you will have
to build your case for disability payments with an array of laboratory
tests and other hard data plus strongly worded, detailed letters from
your physicians attesting to the severity of your disability. Documentation for all medical problems must be complete enough to give the
physician who is part of the SSA evaluation team a clear understanding
of your impairment. In general, CFS patients do best when they apply
for Social Security on the basis of "multiple-system impairment,"
provided they can document a range of body system malfunctions.

Here are hints for assembling a convincing and comprehensive
application to demonstrate to the local disability board of the Social
Security Administration that you have been completely incapacitated
by chronic fatigue syndrome.

- Provide laboratory tests results. Psychometric tests, which measure psychological or cognitive damage, vestibular tests to
  determine the existence of a balance disorder, and tests of sleep
  disorders and immune function have all convinced some disability boards of the legitimacy of a CFS claim. To be sure the
  Social Security board gets all your lab reports, gather them
  together yourself. Hospitals are notorious for slipping on this
  administrative detail and your application can then be denied
  on the grounds of insufficient evidence.

- Letters from your primary-care physicians and any medical
  specialists you see are among the most important pieces of
  substantiating evidence you can present. They should describe
  your case in great detail, citing chapter and verse of your
  medical history to support their statements. Be sure the
  letters indicate how long you have been under a doctor's
  care, the severity and duration of your symptoms, the medical
  tests run prior to diagnosis, and the types of treatment that
  have been tried and how effective they have been. It is important that the letters conclude by stating unequivocally that
  you are 100 percent disabled. If necessary, provide your
  physicians with drafts of the letters you need for their review
  and signature. (Samples are included in *Social Security Disability
  Benefits: How to Get Them, How to Keep Them*, which is listed in
  Appendix C.)

• Ask your employer (past or present) and friends and relatives to write letters for you. An employer willing to describe your past responsibilities and the obvious deterioration in your capacities can provide very effective documentation.

• In characterizing your own disability, include as many specific examples and anecdotes as possible. If you have been keeping a careful log of your condition, provide photocopies as part of your application. Social Security wants to know exactly how your impairment limits function and you'll need to paint a detailed picture for the SSA evaluation team. It is not enough to say simply that you are fatigued or confused. If you had to sit on the sidewalk the last time you ventured outdoors or had to stop driving ever since the afternoon you couldn't remember how to stop the car, say so. Don't overdramatize your condition but don't minimize it either.

• In the required interview, prepare yourself to answer extremely personal questions. A caseworker will be assigned to find out just how your disability affects your daily life and intimate inquiries about your personal habits, love relationships, and household activities are a necessary part of that process.

• Contact your congressional representatives. Although they cannot influence the decision of the Social Security board, their expression of concern will improve the odds of a speedy response and minimize the chance that your application gets lost.

The Appeals Procedure. An initial determination of eligibility is made within 120 days after your Social Security disability claim is filed. No matter how compelling the evidence, a significant number of applicants are initially denied benefits as part of a widespread crackdown on perceived abuses of the system. Like other seriously ill people, many chronic fatigue syndrome patients are ultimately declared eligible for payment, but only after being forced through the hoops of an elaborate appeals process first.

If your request is denied, you may ask for a reconsideration. Although your case will then be independently reviewed by people who were not involved with the initial decision, the chances of a reversal are fairly slim at this stage.

Most successful Social Security disability claims are determined in the next appeals stage, when a case goes before an administrative law judge. This is a face-to-face, private hearing with a judge who has great leeway to make a decision based on subjective criteria. At the hearing, you will have to answer questions from your own attorney, if you have one, and from the judge. You can also call your own witnesses at this hearing. A physician willing to testify can present a compelling case for your eligibility.

If an application is denied by an administration law judge, the Appeals Council of the Social Security Administration makes a final determination on your case. Then claimants have the right to carry appeals into the federal court system. No matter how discouraging the entire process may seem, it is crucial to keep pressing your case because a decision can be reversed at any point, according to Valerie Kistler, a supervisor with a Social Security Administration branch in Boston: "Don't give up hope, keep appealing, keep trying to impress on people how CFS has affected your life."

Although patients may obtain a layer at any time during the application and appeals procedure—and are not obligated to use one at any point—it is generally recommended that you seek counsel by the time a case reaches an administrative law judge. One patient, who ultimately was declared eligible for disability benefits, said that her decision to hire a lawyer was based on practical necessity: "My thinking was so impaired that there was no way I would have been able to cope with all those papers by myself."

Most attorneys who handle Social Security cases accept them on a contingency fee basis, earning no more than 25 percent of past-due benefits if the case is won. If benefits are ultimately denied, the attorney collects no fee although you may be charged for any out-of-pocket expenses incurred. The National Organization for Social Security Claimants Representatives, listed in Appendix B, will refer you to attorneys with special expertise in dealing with the Social Security Administration.

Disability Benefits. If you are declared eligible for Social Security disability benefits, the size of your monthly checks will be determined by your income level and the age and number of your dependents. Some of the benefits may be subject to federal and state taxes. Generally disability checks continue as long as your impairment does but all cases are reviewed periodically. A rather creative aspect of Social Security legislation allows claimants to test their ability to work on a trial basis by continuing to make disability payments for up to nine months—which do not need to be consecutive—after they return to work. For an additional fifteen months, claimants can receive Social Security disability during any month when they cannot work.

After receiving disability checks for twenty-four months, you become eligible for health care coverage under the Medicare program, which is administered by the Health Care Financing Administration (HCFA). Medicare provides no-premium hospital insurance to cover most inpatient hospital care and related health services after leaving the hospital. For a monthly premium, additional insurance is available for doctors' bills and outpatient care.

Other Public Entitlement Programs

A number of other public programs provide benefits to people in need, in some instances whether or not you qualify for Social Security disability payments. Depending on your financial circumstances and work history, some of the following programs could literally prove to be lifesavers.

Supplemental Security Income (SSI). SSI is a federal program supported through general tax revenues. Like the Social Security disability program, it provides a monthly stipend to persons too disabled to work and uses the same medical requirements to determine eligibility. SSI, however, is targeted at individuals with very limited resources and income and does not require any particular work history. Benefit levels are usually lower than Social Security disability payments. SSI recipients cannot also receive Aid to Families with Dependent Children but they are generally eligible for Food Stamps and Medicaid; all three programs are described below. Eligibility for SSI may also entitle an individual to certain homemaker, personal care, or other social support services. An individual on SSI remains eligible for Social Security disability benefits, although those payments generally reduce the size of the SSI check.

Further information about applying for SSI is available from local Social Security offices.

Unemployment Insurance. Each state sets its own criteria for dispensing Unemployment Insurance funds, which are collected via an employer tax. If you have been gainfully employed for a certain period of time (generally about twenty weeks over the past year) and terminated from your job through no fault of your own, you may be eligible to collect Unemployment Insurance benefits. The catch here is that you must also be actively looking for work, a criteria that is likely to exclude many CFS patients, except those who recover quickly.

Further information about applying for Unemployment Insurance is available from the state Department of Labor.

Food Stamps. Food Stamps are generally accepted by grocery stores in lieu of cash for most food items (excluding alcohol and certain ready-to-eat foods). Although the federal government, under the aegis of the U.S. Department of Agriculture, pays for the Food Stamp program, it is administered by state agencies. Eligibility for Food Stamps is based on financial need and takes into consideration the number of people living in a household, household income, and personal assets. Disabled persons can deduct certain expenses from the total income used to determine need if they can prove that those expenses are critical.

Further information about applying for Food Stamps is available through local Social Security offices.

Medicaid. Funded jointly by the federal and state governments, Medicaid is available to low-income people who are unable to pay for the costs of needed medical care. Each state determines its own eligibility criteria and benefit level but strict income and asset limitations apply. In New York, for example, a single person can earn no more than $5,200 annually and maintain reserves in cash or other personal property (excluding the value of a home, furnishings, a car, and clothing) of no more than $3,100. Typically, Medicaid-eligible individuals are also entitled to Food Stamps.

Further information about applying for Medicaid is available from state or county Social Service departments.

Aid to Families with Dependent Children (AFDC). AFDC is available in households with dependent children who are under the age of eighteen or still attending secondary school and living at home. Individuals may be eligible for public assistance if there is no principal wage earner in the household and in some cases if the principal wage earner is unable to work or is unemployed. Strict income and asset restrictions apply. The costs of AFDC programs are shared by federal, state, and local governments with benefit levels determined at the state level. In many states, individuals who are eligible for AFDC are automatically Medicaid-eligible.

Further information about applying for AFDC is available from state or county Social Service departments.

Housing Assistance. Disabled individuals who need to adapt their home by removing architectural barriers, hazards, or other inconvenient features may be eligible for a Title I Home Improvement Loan insured by the U.S. Department of Housing and Urban Development (HUD). Low-income families may also be eligible for housing assistance payments from HUD.

Further information about housing programs benefitting disabled persons is available from the U.S. Department of Housing and Urban Development. HUD has a special advisor on the handicapped in Washington, D.C.

Declaring Bankruptcy

Once upon a time—roughly 450 B.C.—the law allowed a debtor to be put to death so that his body could be carved and divided among his creditors. While a few loansharks may still employ this tactic, our society as a whole has developed rather more civilized ways of dealing with an individual who cannot pay debts. Declaring bankruptcy gives honest debtors an opportunity to wipe clean their slate of financial obligations while providing creditors fair access to remaining assets. Chronic fatigue syndrome patients, who often encounter catastrophic health care costs just when their income has declined precipitously, should be aware of the personal bankruptcy option.

Under the U.S. Constitution, the Congress is specifically empowered to establish uniform laws on personal and corporate bankruptcy and has done so through the Federal Bankruptcy Act. Under this act, an individual is permitted to file a bankruptcy petition in Federal District Court when liabilities exceed income. The use of an attorney, who will undoubtedly require payment in advance, is strongly recommended in this procedure because a number of strategic decisions must be made. New Jersey support group leader Bob Landau, who was forced to declare bankruptcy after a long period of illness, advises patients to plan the move in careful consultation with experts. "There are ways to do it so you won't be completely destitute," notes Landau.

In a bankruptcy proceeding, debtors list total assets and outstanding liabilities and their creditors each file separate claims. Assuming no fraud or concealment of assets is suspected, a court-appointed trustee determines how a debtor's assets will be distributed among all creditors and then discharges remaining debts. State laws sometimes exempt certain personal assets. For example, a debtor may be allowed to keep a primary residence, an automobile, or other personal property deemed indispensable. Once a bankruptcy petition is filed, a paycheck can be protected from garnishment but other payments—including monies currently owed you from an inheritance, a lawsuit, or an outstanding loan—are usually counted among available assets.

Remember a petition for bankruptcy can be filed only once every seven years, tax debt usually cannot be erased, and bankruptcy proceedings deal a severe blow to credit ratings.

Programs for the Disabled

In recent years there has been a clamor of demands from people with a range of physical disabilities who are no longer content to remain isolated from social and economic opportunities. People confined to wheelchairs have demanded that sidewalks, buildings, and public events be made accessible to them; deaf students at Gallaudet University, in Washington, D.C., made history with their successful demands for a deaf president; an insistence on the more careful use of language has helped tear down attitudinal barriers and erase stereotypes.

Much of the impetus for disabled rights comes from Section 504 of the Federal Rehabilitation Act of 1973, which reads, "No otherwise qualified handicapped individual in the United States . . . shall, solely by reason of his handicap, be excluded from the participation in, be denied the benefits of, or be subjected to discrimination under any program of activity receiving federal assistance." Under this legislation, any entity that operates with federal funds must make its programs accessible to persons with a range of disabilities and is barred from employment discrimination.

Although their disabilities are seldom permanent and often invisible, chronic fatigue syndrome patients are entitled to the protections of Section 504. Under the employment provision, for example, an employer has to make reasonable efforts to accommodate someone who needs to rest periodically in order to continue working. Similarly a student suffering from CFS has the legal right to request special arrangements for completing final examinations, rather than having to cram them all into one exhausting week. CFS patients also have access to the grassroots and public sector programs developed for disabled persons in the wake of Section 504, several of which are described below.

Independent Living Centers

Many communities around the country have independent living centers (ILCs), which encourage people with disabilities to maintain self-sufficient and productive lives. Although each center is different, most provide direct services and also work to eliminate some of the societal barriers—be they attitudinal, environmental, social, psychological, or economic—to equal opportunity.

The severe physical disabilities often evident at an independent living center initially startle CFS patients, observes Nancy Durkin, who was executive director of the Center for Independent Living of Southwest Connecticut before she became too ill with chronic fatigue syndrome to continue working. Asking for help from an ILC generally means being willing to define yourself as disabled, which can be difficult for CFS sufferers. But Durkin observes, "If you are at a point of desperation, I can't think of a better resource than the independent living centers. They are a great place to brainstorm different ideas and to make linkages in the community. They know how to help you find peer support and guide you through the system."

Typically ILCs offer information and referral services, assistance in locating accessible and affordable housing, personal care services, peer counseling, and training in skills of adaptive and independent living. Also provided at some centers are opportunities for career development, education, loans, financial counseling, legal advocacy, social and recreational activities, wheelchair-accessible transportation, and services geared to specific disabilities.

Contact one of the national bodies coordinating the activities of the ILC movement, listed in Appendix B, for assistance in locating the independent living center nearest you.

Home-Share Programs

A creative alternative to moving back home with mom and dad—if you are fortunate enough even to have that option—is beginning to receive attention from state Departments on Aging and independent living centers. Called home share or "share a house" programs, they link people who need a place to live with those who have extra space in their houses or apartments and want companionship or additional income from a roommate. Initially developed with the aging population in mind, these programs are also suitable for the chronically ill.

Many different home-sharing arrangements are possible, depending on the needs and wants of both parties. For example, you may be able to strike a deal in which you handle the more sedentary household chores while your roommate agrees to do the grocery shopping and cleaning. Home-share program counselors screen and interview both parties to make sure each gets what they need from the living arrangement.

More information about home-share programs is available from your local Department of Aging or the independent living center in your community.

Library Services

A common complaint of CFS sufferers is an inability to read, either because their concentration is shot or because visual distortions make words appear to dance all over the page. To reduce the tedium and curb the mental atrophy that is part and parcel of the syndrome, CFS patients should know about a special Library of Congress-sponsored loan program. If you are unable to use standard printed materials as a result of a visual or physical impairment, whether it is temporary or permanent, you are eligible to borrow taped books, magazines, reference materials, and music, as well as playback equipment, from participating libraries. All of it can be returned via postage-free mail.

Contact the National Library Service for the Blind and Physically Handicapped, listed in Appendix B, for further information.

Local Programs

Many cities and states offer a variety of other benefits and assistance programs to people with disabilities. Some have strict financial criteria for eligibility whereas others do not. Information about the resources available to chronically ill and disabled people can usually be obtained from the Office of the Mayor or the local Office of the Handicapped in your community.

A few of the most common programs are described below:

- Personal-care attendants. Increasing numbers of states have developed programs through which a disabled individual can hire someone to help with such household chores as cooking, cleaning, or doing the laundry. Eligibility may be based on the nature of the disability, financial need, or both. Because individuals with physical limitations can live independent, productive lives if they have appropriate community support, the availability of personal-care attendants has become one of the core issues in the disabled rights movement.

• Preferential or handicapped parking. Many states provide special license plates or a permit for the car windshield that enables disabled people to park in specially designated—and usually very convenient—parking zones. Individuals who have difficulty walking long distances may want to pick up appropriate application forms at the Department of Motor Vehicles; usually they must be signed by a doctor.

• Subsidized transportation programs. Reduced-fare public transportation is often available for people who meet certain disability criteria. Such programs ease the financial strain borne by disabled persons and also reduce their isolation from mainstream society. Any municipality that receives federal subsidies for their public transit programs is under particular pressure to make their transportation systems more accessible.

• Reduced prices for prescription medicines. A number of states subsidize the cost of prescription medicines, and sometimes other pharmaceutical items. Although states may establish any criteria they wish for eligibility, many make these programs available only to people currently receiving Social Security benefits.

[⌑]

Remaining solvent, obtaining affordable and appropriate health and personal care, and finding emotional support are all crucial components of recovery. But admittedly, these are stopgap measures and most CFS patients are more interested in the prospects for a cure. What's ahead on the research horizon? How can we galvanize Congress and the public health community to make chronic fatigue syndrome a national priority? After reading profiles of more CFS patients, we'll try to answer these questions in the final section of this book.

Profiles: The Patients

Evelyn Eisgram

Evelyn Eisgram has a yard-long résumé: president, Women in the Arts; president, New York Society of Women; board member, Artists' Equity; member, American Society of Contemporary Artists. Her paintings hang in museums and her unique theory of color has sparked curiosity and sometimes heated controversy within the community of artists and earned her a place in the Smithsonian Archives of American Art. But chronic fatigue syndrome has sapped her creative vision and for six long and difficult years she has not painted a stroke.

Eisgram, who looks at least a decade younger than her seventy-three years, is attentive to her appearance and without visible signs of illness. And yet, along with the skepticism that customarily accompanies CFS, she has endured the insulting implication that at her age ill health is simply to be expected—as though her intense exhaustion, panic attacks, dizziness, swollen glands, and the loss of 35 pounds within a month are simply run-of-the-mill symptoms of aging.

Doubts about the legitimacy of her illness spark Eisgram's anger and sometimes stir despair:

> You start to feel that you're some kind of nut. After all these years, there are still people around who think I am a malingerer, a hypochondriac. They'll tell me, "Why don't you forget about it, maybe you're concentrating on it too much" as though I can forget about bumping into walls and having to stop in the middle of the block to take a rest. Patients come to feel that we have to prove ourselves, to show that we are not just hypochondriacs. Maybe it does become an obsession, but it is only because others won't believe us.

Because of her age, physicians have been rigorous in ruling out other diseases. Eisgram has spent a fortune in medical care and sees a gastroenterologist, a cardiac specialist, and a psychiatrist regularly, although she says they have not offered much help. Antidepressants and tranquilizers do provide some relief and the jury is still out on the effectiveness of Shirley Maclaine seminars and crystal-wearing. Despite her commitment to seeking a cure everywhere imaginable, Eisgram says, "I still feel as though I'm pushing a truck uphill."

Bart H.

Wildly colorful flowers enliven the gardens outside Bart's gracious split-level home in the Chicago suburbs. The property abuts a woods and birdhouses are strategically placed about the yard. Inside the decor and furnishings suggest quiet good taste. "None of this is as important to me as good health," says the Chicago dentist, whose activities have been severely curtailed for five years. "If I could exchange it all for a cure, I'd do so tomorrow."

Like many other CFS patients, Bart H. got his first inkling as to the nature of his illness when he ran across an article in the *Annals of Internal Medicine* that proposed the Epstein-Barr virus as the cause of an enigmatic collection of symptoms. "That article described me to a 'T,' " recalls Bart H., who has endured mysterious aches and pains, joint spasms, slurred speech, mood swings, and a kidney disorder over the years. But initial exhilaration about the *Annals* article quickly turned to disappointment when it became clear that more questions than answers remained about the illness. "Most of us care a lot more about treatment than cause. Maybe I'm not being realistic but I keep telling my doctors 'I don't care what it is, just fix it.' "

Bart is less debilitated than some CFS patients and has been able to keep working, although often on a reduced schedule. And he can't do much else. "On the days when I have the energy to take a walk after work, I feel as though I have really accomplished something special. This is major progress to someone with this illness," he says. His inability to predict his strength on any given day has seriously curtailed his social life:

> People really need to understand that we don't have much control over our illness. We can rest up for days to attend a big event and still not be able to make it. The worst thing our friends can do is to suggest that we can do anything we really set our minds to. That's just not the way it is.

Catherine B.

Whether it inspires pangs of patriotism or fond memories of hearty parties, July 4, 1976, has a special ring to most Americans. But to Catherine B., the date is more bitter than sweet, marking the start of an illness that plagues her even now. When the flu-like symptoms first took hold, she was living in London and working as a magazine writer. British doctors were unable to explain her worsening symptoms and she canceled her plans to travel to Europe in favor of an early return to the United States.

It was to be another ten years before a firm diagnosis of chronic fatigue syndrome was made. "It took a long time for me to realize this was something more than just my constitution being on the meager side," says Catherine, who has learned to accept and live with her reduced energy levels better than many people. Nonetheless, having what she calls a "smaller window of good times" has been very frustrating professionally. Now a free-lance travel writer, Catherine B. believes she has had no more than "half a career" because of the limitations imposed on her by CFS. "I have to be very conservative about what I can take on," she says. "I know I'm not a powerhouse, I can't get oodles of things done in a short time. Naps are very much a part of my life and I just work whenever I can."

A particularly sensitive issue for Catherine has been the challenge of coping with chronic illness in the context of a marriage. "My husband is very energetic. He can work twelve or fourteen hours a day and then be ready to go out. My not going out cut down considerably on his socializing and this used to be a serious area of contention for us." Candid discussion and a willingness on the part of both parties to compromise finally helped resolve the problem, with the couple opting for greater independence. Says Catherine: "Now that we are old and wiser, we've realized that couples don't always have to lead the same lives, you don't have to do everything together. In the long run, his having so much energy makes my life easier—we balance each other out."

As the leader of a patient support group in Manhattan, Catherine B. is part of a nationwide movement to bring public attention and funding to the problem of CFS. "I view the support group as a political tool," she says. Admittedly, her motives aren't entirely altruistic:

> If the group is well-organized and helps make the disease visible to grant makers, the government, and the drug companies, then research will be done. If research is done, it is possible that therapies will be developed. And if therapies are developed, it is possible that I will feel better.

Morty R.

Morty R., age fifty-two, is a familiar figure on the world-class stages of New York City, Chicago, New Haven, Minneapolis, Philadelphia, Boston, and elsewhere. A member of Actor's Equity for twenty years, he is known to television audiences for his work on seventy television shows. But few people know Morty suffers from chronic fatigue syndrome.

Illness set in suddenly, shortly after he had begun rehearsals for his latest Broadway play. "It hit me like a ton of bricks," Morty recalls. "All of a sudden my legs literally wouldn't work. They just felt totally worn out. That same day I banged my leg against a table and watched a black-and-blue mark spread wildly across my shin." Within a few months he had lost so much weight that a close friend told him, "If you hadn't been with your son, I wouldn't have recognized you. You look like a pencil."

In his search for an appropriate diagnosis, Morty was tested for the AIDS virus, tuberculosis, and a slew of other terrifying diseases. The results were all negative. Only his Epstein-Barr virus titers were abnormally high, a finding made only after Morty insisted that his doctor run the test. Four years after being given a name for his disquieting collection of symptoms, Morty continues to suffer from an exhaustion that no amount of sleep will cure. He still bruises easily, often finds it hard to catch his breath, and sometimes suffers from night sweats.

The effect on his career generates enormous stress for the actor. "I don't think I'd get hired if a director knew I was sick. He'll hesitate and probably say, 'I'd like to use him but I understand he is sick and I just can't take the chance." So Morty keeps silent about the illness that has left him feeling drugged much of the time but every performance is a struggle and most of his spare time is spent in bed. "I'm not going to be able to go on like this much longer," says Morty R. "The energy it takes to be onstage is extraordinary. But the idea of giving up acting is terrifying to me."

PART IV

The Future

9

■

On the Frontlines:
Research Directions and
Patient Advocacy Work
for Tomorrow

I'm convinced this is a real disease, I know these people are suffering. Because of AIDS, this thing has been put on the back burner, it hasn't gotten the attention it deserves. That's why we're so far behind. What we need is the dissemination of accurate information and good controlled medical studies. It should not be that difficult to find out the cause of chronic fatigue syndrome and what treatments work.

—Dr. Neil Singer, San Francisco, California

Considering all the research now going on, I think we are going to see a major breakthrough in chronic fatigue syndrome.

—Dr. Richard DuBois, Atlanta Medical Associates,
Atlanta, Georgia

Until the Centers for Disease Control issued its working definition of chronic fatigue syndrome in spring 1988, researchers could not be certain that the same set of criteria was being used to evaluate patients. Questions about the credibility of the CFS diagnosis lingered and many physicians harbored a suspicion that their patients were simply stressed-out or depressed.

Now, thanks in large measure to the tenacity of CFS patients themselves, to a handful of dedicated physicians and researchers, and to a probing press, the illness has begun to receive the serious scrutiny it deserves. Epidemiological studies that will provide a reliable head count of CFS patients are underway. Scientists at the nation's most prestigious public and private research institutions and universities— including the National Institutes of Health, Harvard Medical Center, the School of Public Health at Yale University, the San Francisco and Los Angeles branches of the University of California, the University of North Carolina at Chapel Hill, Pittsburgh Cancer Institute, the National Jewish Center of Immunology and Respiratory Medicine, and New York City's Mount Sinai Hospital, to name but a few—have turned their attention to the syndrome. Support groups have sprung up around the country to ease the isolation and fear that many patients have suffered in the past.

One of the most exciting developments on the horizon is the growing organizational strength of the National Chronic Fatigue Syndrome Advisory Council, a high-level body of clinicians and researchers. Dr. Anthony Komaroff, Chief of the Division of General Medicine at Boston's Brigham and Women's Hospital, is council president. Dr. Paul Cheney, senior staff physician in the Department of General Internal Medicine at the Nalle Clinic, is vice president. Active participation is also expected from patient advocate groups. The council is striving to improve information dissemination, expand CFS research, set gold standards for laboratory testing, and encourage medical colleagues to become more actively involved in CFS research.

But an enormous amount of work remains to be done. Reaching diagnosis still involves guesswork and the time-consuming, costly process of excluding other diseases. We don't understand what causes CFS, we can't cure it, and treatment options are inadequate. And, as if to add insult to a patient's already injured life, we have yet to create a health care system that guarantees access to affordable care: Right now, those too ill to work stand to lose their health insurance.

The nightmare of chronic fatigue syndrome has not ended but the dawn of a new day draws nearer. Despite the litany of unknowns, scientific investigation into CFS is going forward at a quickening clip. Increasing numbers of physicians are accepting the syndrome as a real, albeit enigmatic, illness. Political activism has grown at both the local and federal levels, empowering patients with a sense of control over their lives while guaranteeing that public officials will feel pressure to allocate adequate resources to combat CFS.

New Directions in Research

When asked about the research still needed in the area of chronic fatigue syndrome, internist Dr. Carol Jessop rolled her eyes in dismay and answered with a single word: "Lots." Primary-care physicians suffer most keenly from the dearth of laboratory tests that make a CFS diagnosis definitive, as well as from the limitations of treatment and the poor understanding of cause. They are also concerned about the possibility that CFS is a risk factor for other diseases. "We need to find out the relationship between CFS and AIDS or malignancy, if there is any, so that we can provide appropriate screening to CFS patients during the course of their illness and beyond," says Dr. Jessop.

Epidemiologists like Dr. Paul Levine of the National Cancer Institute, who is studying the incidence and pattern of the illness, need to know whether reported CFS epidemics represent a recurrence of precisely the same event or a series of clinically indistinguishable events with different causes. "Outbreaks have been reported for decades but it is hard to know if we are comparing the same phenomena," says Dr. Levine. "What we really need to do is identify a new cluster as it is occurring and go in and study that population. Then we can use a very strict case definition and really pinpoint the abnormalities."

One of the scientists helping chart the directions of future CFS research is Dr. Nathaniel Brown, who chaired an ad-hoc committee reviewing CFS research proposals submitted to the National Institutes of Health. From his offices at the sprawling North Shore University Hospital on Long Island, where he is a pediatric infectious disease specialist, Brown talks about the three broad areas where he believes further research into chronic fatigue syndrome is most urgently needed:

- First, detection and surveillance of CFS should be expanded and the Centers for Disease Control's existing case definition should be improved. Within this category, controlled studies for alleged risk factors—viral and otherwise—are particularly crucial. According to Brown, some of the early studies, particularly those prior to the CDC definition, lacked proper controls and failed to meet the rigorous criteria that assures scientific validity.

- Second, more information is needed about the latency and reactivation of persistent viruses and how they interact with the body's cytokines, the cell-signaling protein molecules that are a crucial part of appropriate immune responses.

• Third, a more sophisticated understanding of neuroimmunology and the neurophysiology of stress is vital. Simply put, this means sharpening our knowledge of the interaction between the immune system and the nervous system, a field of study made possible only because of the explosive growth of scientific knowledge. "In the past it has been difficult to do meaningful research in this area because both systems are very complicated and we didn't really have a good handle on either one. In the past five or ten years, we have made incredible progress," Brown says.

Any knowledge that can be gathered about chronic fatigue syndrome is likely to have multiple paybacks, expanding our understanding of the immune system, the physiological effects of stress, the nature of autoimmunity, and the role of genetic predisposition in disease. "You can't go wrong pouring funds into chronic fatigue syndrome because we'll get our money's worth out of the studies," says Dr. Paul Cheney, noting that the syndrome's complexity makes it a very fertile area of ground-breaking research.

The Washington Scene

In 1988, the U.S. Congress took three measures that together sent a message to the nation that chronic fatigue syndrome had finally assumed a place of importance on the public health agenda: First, it allocated $1.2 million, plus the equivalent of eight full-time jobs, to epidemiological studies underway at the Centers for Disease Control. Second, it urged the National Institutes of Health to continue to expand its biomedical research on chronic fatigue syndrome, with particular emphasis on the interplay between CFS and viruses, the immune system, and AIDS. And third, it instructed the Social Security Administration to establish more uniform criteria for granting disability payments to chronic fatigue syndrome patients.

Congressional appropriations continued to grow and by fiscal year 1992, patient groups were seeking $2.8 million to allow the Centers for Disease Control to continue its four-city surveillance study and expand it to include children. Much of the credit for congressional interest in chronic fatigue syndrome rests with two savvy men whose lives were changed by the illness. Barry Sleight, a lifelong resident of Washington, D.C., is a patient. Theodore van Zelst, who runs Minnan, a small family foundation near Chicago, is the father of one. Convinced that without federal funds, CFS research would progress at a snail's pace amid lingering skepticism from the medical community, each became skillful at maneuvering through the federal bureaucracy and articulate in their efforts to galvanize Congress into action. Together they are a force to be reckoned with on Capitol Hill.

Van Zelst first gave stirring testimony before congressional appropriations committees in 1984 and has done so every year since then. As executive director of the Chronic Fatigue Syndrome Institute, a patient advocacy group, Sleight also gives testimony and speaks with hundreds of congressional representatives, their staff, and members of the public health community in order to increase understanding of CFS and push for reasonable funding levels. He knows how to hit a nerve with cost-conscious public officials: In recent testimony he said, "Our society is already paying social and economic costs of this disease such as lost jobs, broken homes, lost productivity, lost tax receipts, bankruptcies, and increased health care and disability costs."

While congressional interest in chronic fatigue syndrome and how it affects their constituencies has come a long way in recent years, additional appropriations will be needed. Citizen participation is crucial to keeping elected representatives committed to CFS. "Congress begins to pay attention to an illness when representatives get inquiries about it from their constituency and when it begins to occupy staff time," says Barry Sleight, who is convinced that the cards, letters, and telephone calls that have poured into congressional offices from concerned patients forced lawmakers to take note.

As a taxpayer and a voter, your efforts make an important difference. Let your senators and congressmen know that you are out there—and that you are watching to see how they respond to CFS funding requests. Urge your friends and family to do the same. A brief note urging increased allocations for chronic fatigue syndrome is a good start. Better yet, send detailed and personal letters describing your own involvement with the illness and how your experiences highlight the need for better diagnostic and treatment methods. Follow up your letters with phone calls or a telegram. Don't ease up on the pressure. And remind your congressional representatives that your vote on election day depends on their votes for CFS research funds.

Local Organizing:
The Art of Gentle Persuasion

While medical research is traditionally funded largely at the federal level, a great deal of responsibility for patient care and public education rests with local communities. Local organizers accross the country are working to educate public health departments and elected officials about CFS and to urge them to put resources into patient tracking, public education, physician referral, and other needed tasks.

The San Francisco Model

An important model for local activists has emerged in San Francisco. Credit for the work in the Bay Area belongs largely to Jan Montgomery. A strong feminist, she was a professional fund-raiser and political organizer before suddenly falling ill in 1984. Although her symptoms continue to wax and wane, she established the Chronic Fatigue and Immune Dysfunction Foundation, based in the Bay Area, as a tool of political advocacy and fund-raising. "This issue chose me," she explains somewhat grimly. "If you were in Germany during the war, you didn't get to pick your issue, yet there was no greater test of leadership."

Shortly before she became ill, Montgomery had been tapped to run the reelection campaign of San Francisco Supervisor Nancy Walker. Although her bout with CFS nipped that appointment in the bud, the fortuitous friendship helped speed the credibility with which the syndrome has been received in that wild but gracious city some call Baghdad by the Bay. Because Walker knew Montgomery and believed she was sick, the supervisor helped her assemble an organizing group and saw that she had unusually generous access to the city's most influential leaders.

"Our basic strategy is to think globally and act locally," says the dynamic Montgomery.

> What works is knowing who is influential and getting them to pick up this issue as part of their political agenda. We tell our story and we hope that they will start telling it to others. Just having a critical mass of participation is going to make things happen.

Montgomery's group has met with scores of city, state, and public health officials to talk about CFS and to plead for funds. In a community still reeling from the impact of AIDS, the reaction to her efforts has, predictably, been mixed. Overwhelmed by the demands of the AIDS epidemic, some public officials have turned a deaf ear, evidently hoping that this latest assault will simply vanish. Others, though, have been more responsive, determined perhaps to avoid the mistakes made when the AIDS crisis first came to light.

As a result, a CFS task force has been assembled with representatives from the Mayor's Office, the city Health Department, community clinics, and AIDS-related organizations. Local funds have been committed to track the incidence of chronic fatigue syndrome, physician and patient surveys are underway, physician referral lists are being compiled, and a major scientific conference was held in the spring of 1989. These activities put San Francisco well ahead of most other communities, where the public health impact of the illness has only recently been recognized.

Tips for Organizing at Home

Here are some hints on local organizing, distilled from ongoing work in San Francisco and elsewhere:

- Before getting stared, find people skilled in the art of political organizing and seek their advice and counsel. There's no sense in reinventing the wheel when there are folks out there who already know how it spins. In San Francisco, for example, Jan Montgomery brainstormed with the San Francisco AIDS Foundation, which has been highly effective in garnering funds for AIDS services.

- Determine a political agenda that is appropriate to your community and identify elected and appointed officials with the power to respond to that agenda. Individuals who can influence health policies are most often found in the local public health department; on local governing bodies, such as city councils or boards of supervisors; and on citizen committees and volunteer organizations.

- Personal connections are always the best way to attract attention from the powerful. Make the right contacts by talking with everyone you know: Someone is sure to know someone who knows someone who can introduce you to someone. Press for meetings in which you can explain the nature of chronic fatigue syndrome and the importance of responding to it in a timely and responsible manner.

- Be as specific as possible in making your requests. Some things to ask for are help in educating the public about CFS; epidemiological surveys to nail down the extent of the problem locally; a conference for physicians and public health officials to keep them current on research developments; and specialized clinics to ensure appropriate treatment for patients. Follow up these requests with letter-writing campaigns and reminder phone calls to reinforce your message; it is important that public officials know their constituency is deeply concerned about this issue.

- Enlist the support of healthy people in your organizing efforts. This support is crucial not only because the energy of CFS patients is understandably limited but because it adds weight and credibility to your cause.

- Consider other ways to spread the word about chronic fatigue syndrome in your community. If there is a university in the area, try to interest scientists and health policy specialists in CFS-related research. Contact local professional associations of physicians, nurses, or public health workers and be certain they are up to date on the latest medical information. Link up with other patient organizations with whom you share common concerns to create the empowering strength of numbers.

Become a Fund-raiser

A number of CFS-related fund-raising activities are taking place around the country—to build links among local support groups, to underwrite scientific research, and to fund advocacy work in Washington, D.C. Details are available from many of the CFS organizations listed in Appendix B.

Whether you wish to participate in nationwide projects or concentrate on local support work, here are some guidelines for raising funds in your community:

- Educate your friends, family, employers, and neighbors about CFS. People need to understand a cause before they will donate to it. Don't think of fund-raising as asking for a handout. View it as providing an opportunity for those who care about you to do something tangible on your behalf.

- Write letters to everyone you can think of describing chronic fatigue syndrome and explaining how it has personally affected you. Then ask for contributions toward ongoing research and advocacy work. Provide names and addresses of specific CFS projects sponsored through nonprofit institutions (make sure they have 501(c) (3) tax status), let your friends and family know exactly how their funds will be used, and remind them that all contributions are tax-deductible.

- Talk with your employers and co-workers about how they can help. Many companies have special gift programs in which they match the contributions made by employees. One persuasive argument to use while soliciting donations for chronic fatigue syndrome from employers is that the illness costs them a lot of money in sicktime pay and in the loss of valued employees.

[   ]

While much medical research remains undone and the patchwork system of emotional, social, and financial supports is still inadequate for many patients, the struggle to understand chronic fatigue syndrome has come a long way in a relatively short time. Despite shoestring budgets and the strain of illness, patients groups have developed a strong voice in their local communities and an influential presence in Washington. Lawmakers, physicians, scientists, and even the decision makers at the Social Security Administration have all taken note and are beginning to respond appropriately. "We don't have the resources to have big dinners, receptions, golf club dates, or sailboat trips," said political organizer Barry Sleight at a fund-raising event. "We have to appeal to the heart, remind our elected representatives that there are people suffering out there."

Appendix A:
How the Centers for Disease
Control Defines CFS

In spring 1988, the Centers for Disease Control, the Atlanta-based federal public health agency, published an official definition of chronic fatigue syndrome. The move was widely hailed as an acknowledgement of CFS's legitimacy and as an important step toward broadening scientific understanding of CFS.

Major Criteria

According to the Centers for Disease Control, a case of chronic fatigue syndrome must fulfill these two major criteria:

1. New onset of persistent or relapsing, debilitating fatigue or easy fatigability in a person who has no previous history of similar symptoms. The fatigue does not resolve with bed rest and is severe enough to reduce or impair average daily activity below 50 percent of the patient's customary level for at least six months.

2. Other clinical conditions that may produce similar symptoms must be excluded by thorough evaluation, based on a medical history, physical examination, and appropriate laboratory tests. Conditions specifically mentioned by the CDC include malignancy; autoimmune diseases; localized infection; chronic or subacute bacterial, fungal, or parasite disease (such as Lyme disease, tuberculosis, toxoplasmosis, amebas, or giardia); AIDS, AIDS-related condition (ARC) or any other HIV-related infection; chronic psychiatric disease (such as depression, neurosis, schizophrenia); chronic use of tranquilizers, drug dependency

or abuse; side effects of medication or a toxic agent (such as a chemical solvent or a pesticide); chronic inflammatory disease; neuromuscular disease, such as multiple sclerosis or myasthenia gravis; endocrine disease, such as hypothyroidism or diabetes; any other known chronic pulmonary, renal, cardiac, hepatic (relating to the liver), or hematologic (relating to blood or blood-forming tissues) disease.

Minor Criteria

In addition to fulfilling both major criteria, the CDC requires that patients report six or more of the following symptoms *plus* two or more of the following physical signs (or just eight or more of the symptoms).

Symptom Criteria

Relevant symptoms must have begun at the time fatigue set in, or afterward and persisted or recurred over a period of six months:

1. Mild fever (between 37.5°C and 38.6°C or between 99.5°F and 101.48°F when taken orally by the patient) or chills

2. Sore throat

3. Painful lymph nodes

4. Unexplained, generalized muscle weakness

5. Muscle discomfort or pain

6. Generalized fatigue lasting twenty-four hours or more after a level of exercise that would have been easily tolerated prior to illness

7. Headaches that differ in type or severity from those prior to illness

8. Severe joint pain without joint swelling or redness

9. At least one neuropsychological complaint, such as excessive irritability, confusion, inability to concentrate, depression, difficulty thinking, photophobia, forgetfulness, or impaired vision

10. Sleep disturbances

11. Rapid onset within a few hours or a few days, of above symptoms

Physical Criteria

Relevant physical signs must be documented by a physician on at least two occasions, at least one month apart:

1. Low-grade fever (orally, between 37.5°C and 38.6°C or between 99.5°F and 101.48°F; rectally, between 37.8°C and 38.8°C or between 100.4°F and 101.84°F)

2. Inflammation of the mucous membranes, throat, or upper respiratory tract, without pus in the secretions

3. Palpable or tender lymph nodes

This definition was first published in the March 1988 issue of *Annals of Internal Medicine.* A reprint of that article is available from Dr. Gary P. Holmes, Division of Viral Diseases, Center for Infectious Diseases, Centers for Disease Control, Atlanta, Georgia 30333.

Appendix B:
Resources

The CFS/CFIDS Support Network

The three national organizations of the CFS/CFIDS Support Network can provide lists of local support groups in your area, make physician referrals, and provide practical and emotional support to patients. In addition, each of these organizations encourages research and political advocacy, disseminates information to health professionals, publishes a newsletter, and strives to obtain more media coverage for the illness.

Chronic Fatigue Immune Dysfunction Syndrome Society
P.O. Box 230108
Portland, Oregon 97223
(503) 684-5261
Yvonne Alderman, Office Manager

Chronic Fatigue and Immune Dysfunction Syndrome Association
P.O. Box 220398
Charlotte, North Carolina 28222
(800) 44-CFIDS and (900) 988-CFID
Marc Iverson, President
Kim Kenney, Director of Operations

National Chronic Fatigue Syndrome Association
3521 Broadway, Suite 222
Kansas City, Missouri 64111
(816) 931-4777
Janet Bohanon, Orvalene Prewitt, Co-Directors

Several other CFS/CFIDS organizations also make valuable contributions to organizing and support group activities:

183

National Chronic Fatigue Syndrome Advisory Council
Corresponding Office: 12106 E. 54th Terrace
Kansas City, Missouri 64133
Dr. Anthony Komaroff, Council President
An association of physicians, researchers, and patients who have joined forces to improve access to accurate information about chronic fatigue syndrome. The organization also seeks to expand research funding for the illness.

MINNAN, Inc.
P.O. Box 582
Glenview, Illinois 60025
Theodore Van Zelst, Director
A 30-year-old private foundation that is active in the fields of health and education, MINNAN has provided financial support to CFS research studies since 1984. The organization is also involved in CFS advocacy work, tracking federal developments relating to CFS, and giving testimony to congressional appropriations committees.

Chronic Fatigue Immune Dysfunction Syndrome Foundation
965 Mission St., Suite 425
San Francisco, California 94103
(415) 882-9986
Jan Montgomery, Director
Works to involve San Francisco public officials in tracking the incidence of chronic fatigue syndrome and gaining recognition for it as a public health priority. The foundation also fields press inquiries, works with organizations involved in other health policy and human rights issues, and helps train individuals and groups to build political support in their communities.

United Federation of CFS/CFIDS/CEBV Organizations
Box 14603
Tucson, Arizona 85732
(602) 298-8627
Larry A. Sakin, Chair
An association that aims to improve communication among patient support groups around the country.

CFIDS Action Campaign for the United States (CACTUS)
c/o CFIDS Foundation
965 Market Street, Suite 425
San Francisco, California 94103
(415) 882-9986

A coalition of activists dedicated to patient empowerment, expanding public funding for support services and research, improved media coverage of CFIDS, and collaboration with other activists health organizations.

CFS Computer Bulletin Board

Chronic fatigue syndrome goes high-tech with two on-line bulletin boards (in Massachusetts and Arizona).

Called the USA CFIDS/CFS BBS, it uses the WILDCAT! BBS program, and can be reached at (508) 468-6208. The modem specifications are 8 bit word, and no parity, one stop bit (8/n/1) at 300, 1200 or 2400 baud. Operating hours are: noon to midnight, seven days a week. The second electronic service is targeted mostly at researchers and physicians and it's called Tucson CFS BBS. Modem specifications: 8 data bits, no parity, 1 stop bit, full duplex. Up to 2400 baud. Telephone: (602) 749-0040.

Specialized Medical Services

The following clinics specialize in the treatment of chronic fatigue syndrome patients. A number of other clinics are under development around the country; contact your local support group or the national associations for further information.

Chronic Fatigue and Immune Disorder Center
7800 Fannin
Houston, Texas 77054
(713) 790-9680
Dr. Patricia Salvato, Medical Director

Chronic Fatigue Syndrome Institute
500 South Anaheim Hills Road
Suite 128
Anaheim Hills, California 92807
(714) 998-2780
Dr. Jay Goldstein, Director

International CFS Organizations

The patient support group work abroad, which has been ongoing since 1980, created the models for much of the activity in the United States. CFS is usually called myalgic encephalomyelitis (ME) overseas, but scientists have become increasingly certain that both terms describe the same ailment. The largest organizations are the ME Society in England and the ANZME Society in Australia and New Zealand; other groups are also listed below.

Australian & New Zealand Myalgic Encephalomyelitis Society (ANZME)
P.O. Box 35-429
Browns Bay
Auckland 10, New Zealand
Contact: Jim Brookchurch

Myalgic Encephalomyelitis Association of Canada
1301 Plante Drive
Ottawa, Ontario, Canada
Contact: Rod Blaker

Canada CFS Information
154 Timberline Trail
Aurora, Ontario L4G5Z5, Canada
Contact: Ann Teehan

Myalgic Encephalomyelitis Association
Box 8
Stanford-le-Hope
Essex SS17 8EX, England
Contact: Peter M. Blackman

Dutch Myalgic Encephalomyelitis Foundation
M. E. Stichting
Postbus 23670
11000 ED Amsterdam ZO, Holland
Contact: Marion Lescrauwaet

Hong Kong ME Information
60B Conduit Road, 3rd Floor
Hong Kong
Contact: D. Edwards

Papua, New Guinea Myalgic Encephalomyelitis Support
Box 44
Ukarumpa, Via Lac, Papua, New Guinea

ME Awareness Group
66 Third St.
Lower Houghton, 2198 South Africa
Contact: Janine Shawell

Related Resources for CFS Patients

American Academy for Environmental Medicine
Box 16106
Denver, Colorado 80216
The Academy provides information about the field of clinical
ecology, the study of allergic reactions to substances in the environ-
ment, and the range of chronic diseases they are alleged to cause.
Referrals to practitioners are available.

Association of Professional Sleep Societies (APSS)
604 Second Street, S.W.
Rochester, Minnesota 55902
Accredits sleep clinics around the country and offers consumer
information on sleep disorders. APSS has a directory available listing
its accredited sleep clinics.

Asthma and Allergy Foundation of America
1717 Massachusetts Avenue, N.W.
Suite 305
Washington, D.C. 20036
(202) 265-0265 or (800) 7-ASTHMA
Dedicated to finding a cure for asthma and other allergic disorders and providing patient education, research, and service
programs.

Division of Viral Diseases
Center for Infectious Diseases
Centers for Disease Control
Atlanta, Georgia 30333
(404) 332-4555
The Centers for Disease Control, the federal agency charged with monitoring the public health, has embarked on a major epidemiological study of chronic fatigue syndrome. Further background is available from the above address.

Clearinghouse on Disability Information
Office of Special Education and Rehabilitative Services
U.S. Department of Education
Room 3132, Switzer Building
Washington, D.C. 20202
(202) 732-1723
Created by the Rehabilitation Act of 1973, the Clearinghouse on Disability Information is a centralized source of information about federal, state, and local programs for disabled persons. It also tracks relevant legislation and makes appropriate referrals. Publications available: "OSERS News in Print," a newsletter on federal activities affecting people with disabilities; "Pocket Guide to Federal Help for Individuals with Disabilities"; and "A Summary of Existing Legislation Affecting Persons with Disabilities."

Vestibular and Balance Disorders Association of America
1015 N.W. 22nd Avenue
Portland, Oregon 97210
(503) 229-7705
Joan Darling, Managing Director
An information and support organization for people coping with dizziness, balance disorders, and related hearing problems. A number of publications, including a quarterly newsletter, On the Level, are available.

Independent Living Research Utilization
2323 South Shepherd Street, Suite 1000
Houston, Texas
(713) 520-0232
TDD: 520-5136
Federally funded research and training center that maintains a computerized registry of independent living centers and similar pro-

grams around the country. ILCs help people with disabilities maintain self-sufficient and productive lives within their own communities and generally offer information and referral services, peer counseling, and training in skills of independent living and advocacy.

National Council on Independent Living
Troy Atrium, Fourth St. and Broadway
Troy, NY 12180
Denise Figueroa, President
(518) 274-1979
Founded in 1982, the National Council on Independent Living works to strengthen the movement for independent living with technical assistance, public education, and legislative advocacy. The council can also make referrals to local independent living centers.

National Institute of Allergy and Infectious Diseases (NIAID)
Office of Communications
9000 Rockville Pike
Building 31, Room 7A32
Bethesda, Maryland 20892
(301) 496-5717
NIAID, a branch of the National Institutes of Health, has been bombarded with inquiries from CFS patients. Researchers at the institute are monitoring a number of patients over a period of several years to see how their condition changes and are also conducting experimental drug trials. An informational background piece on chronic fatigue syndrome is available from NIAID.

National Organization for Rare Disorders (NORD)
Box 8923
New Fairfield, Connecticut 06812-1783
(203) 746-6518
NORD links 150 different disease-focused organizations in order to maximize their visibility and access to research funds. The organization also publishes a newsletter, the *Orphan Disease Update*, and maintains a rare disease data base, which can be accessed via CompuServe on a personal computer (at the prompt, type "Go RDB" or "Go NORD").

National Organization of Social Security Claimants'
Representatives (NOSSCR)
19 East Central Avenue
Pearl River, New York 10965
(800) 431-2804
(914) 735-8812
NOSSCR is a membership organization of attorneys who represent individuals applying for Social Security disability or SSI. They will answer questions about the application and appeals process and make referrals to local attorneys.

Libraries

Center for Medical Consumers
237 Thomson Street
New York, New York 10012
(212) 674-7105

Plane Tree Health Resource Center
2040 Webster Street
San Francisco, California 94115
(415) 707-3680
Both libraries operate on the premise that consumers need access to current information in order to make informed choices about their health. Current medical literature is clipped and filed by subject and books are available on many different topics. Staff is knowledgeable and helpful.

National Library Service for the Blind and Physically Handicapped
Library of Congress
1291 Taylor St., N.W.
Washington, D.C. 20542
(202) 287-5100
In cooperation with a network of regional libraries, the Library of Congress provides free loans to persons who are unable to read or use standard printed materials because of a visual or physical impairment. An extensive collection of books, magazines, bibliographies, directories, and reference circulars are available and can be delivered and returned by postage-free mail.
Contact the National Library Service for the Blind and Physically Handicapped for a list of available publications and the participating libraries in your area.

Appendix C:
Key Reading

Articles

In recent years, hundreds of articles about chronic fatigue syndrome have appeared in newspapers and magazines around the country. Television stations have also picked up the story, with special pieces appearing on such programs as "Nightline" and "20/20." The CFIDS Society in Portland, Oregon maintains extensive bibliography listings and the CFIDS Association in Charlotte, North Carolina summarizes new articles in its monthly newsletter. A few key articles are described here. (Because of the confusion surrounding the appropriate name for this disorder, many of these articles still call it chronic Epstein-Barr virus infection or chronic mononucleosis.)

Popular Press

Some of the best articles to provide a general background about chronic fatigue syndrome are as follows:

"Chronic Fatigue Syndrome Finally Gets Some Respect." By Lawrence K. Altman. *New York Times*. December 4, 1990.

"Chronic Fatigue Syndrome: A Debilitating Disease Afflicts Millions—and the Cause is Still a Mystery." Cover story. *Newsweek*. November 12, 1990.

"Chronic Fatigue: All in the Mind?" *Consumer Reports*. October 1990.

"Mysterious Malaise." By Paul Weingarten. *Chicago Tribune*. October 21, 1990.

"Chronic Fatigue Gains Credibility." By Kim Painter. *USA Today*. September 18, 1990.

"Chronic Fatigue Syndrome: How to Recognize It and What to Do About It." By Jane E. Brody. *New York Times*, July 28, 1988.

"Yuppie Flu: Do You Have It?" By Leanne Kleinmann. *Health*, April 1988.

"Newest Mystery Illness: Chronic Fatigue Syndrome." By Linda Marsa.
    Redbook, April 1988.
"A Baffling Syndrome, Perhaps Born of Stress, Leaves a Would-Be
    Screenwriter Sick and Tired." By Lyn Hemmerdinger. *People*,
    April 25, 1988.
"A Special Report on Epstein-Barr Viral Syndrome." By Annie Stuart.
    Medical Selfcare, November/December 1987.
"Journey into Fear: The Growing Nightmare of Epstein-Barr Virus."
    By Hillary Johnson. *Rolling Stone*, July 30, 1987 and August 13,
    1987 (Parts I and II).
"Raggedy Ann Town." By William Boly. *Hippocrates*, July/August
    1987.

Medical Journals

Although some of these articles are rather technical for the lay
reader, they are important to an understanding of current scientific
thinking about the syndrome:

"Retroviral sequences related to human T-lymphotropic virus type II
    in patients with Chronic Fatigue Immune Dysfunction Syndrome."
    By Elaine DeFreitas et al. *Proceedings of the National Academy of
    Science*, Vol. 88. April 1991.
Study concludes there is an association between CFIDS and HTLV-II,
a retrovirus in the same family as AIDS.

"Prevalence of Chronic Fatigue Syndrome in an Australian Popula-
    tion." By Andrew R. Lloyd et al. *The Medical Journal of Australia*,
    Vol. 153. November 5, 1990.
Epidemiological study detected 42 patients with CFS in a population
of 114,000. The mean age at onset of symptoms was almost twenty-
nine and symptoms typically lasted for thirty months. There was no
correlation with class status and only slightly more women than men
were afflicted.

"Immunologic Abnormalities in Chronic Fatigue Syndrome." By Nancy
    G. Klimas et al. *Journal of Clinical Microbiology*. June 1990.
Subjects studied were found to have multiple immunologic abnormalities as detected by laboratory markers.

"Chronic Fatigue Syndrome: Medicine for the Public." June 1990.
    "Chronic Fatigue Syndrome: A Pamphlet for Physicians." October
    1990. By the National Institute of Allergy and Infectious Diseases.

Overviews for both health care providers and patients. Among the topics discussed: the course of the illness, its prevalence in the population, its connection with depression, and possible causes, with a particular emphasis on immune system abnormalities.

"The Psychiatric Status of Patients with the Chronic Fatigue Syndrome." By Ian Hickie et al. *British Journal of Psychiatry*, Vol. 156. 1990.
Psychological disturbances among patients with chronic fatigue syndrome are found to be a consequence, rather than a cause, of the syndrome.

"Chronic Fatigue: Taking the Syndrome Seriously." By Mitchel L. Zoler. *Medical World News*, December 12, 1988.
Discussion of the medical community's evolving interest in CFS, the controversy over the Centers for Disease Control's clinical definition, and the directions of future research.

"The Frequency of the Chronic Fatigue Syndrome in Patients with Symptoms of Persistent Fatigue." By Peter Manu et al. *Annals of Internal Medicine*, October 1, 1988.
Authors look at a sample of fatigued individuals and conclude that only 5 percent met the CDC criteria for chronic fatigue syndrome and that many of the rest suffer from psychiatric disorders.

"Chronic Fatigue Syndrome: A Working Case Definition." By Dr. Gary Holmes et al. *Annals of Internal Medicine*, March 1988.
Official Centers for Disease Control definition of chronic fatigue syndrome, which finally enables researchers to be certain they are examining the same patient population.

"Chronic Mononucleosis Syndrome." By Dr. Stephen E. Straus. *Journal of Infectious Diseases*, March 1988.
Excellent overview of research to date. Author reviews major published studies, proposes diagnostic criteria, discusses links with depression, and describes distinctive immunological features.

"Chronic Mononucleosis—It Almost Never Happens." By Dr. Edwin J. Jacobson.
"Chronic Mononucleosis—A Legitimate Diagnosis." By Dr. Martin Tobi and Dr. Stephen E. Straus. *Postgraduate Medicine*, January 1988.
In these two articles, physicians debate the legitimacy of the chronic mononucleosis diagnosis. Jacobson says evidence does not suggest a

viral cause for the illness; Tobi and Straus say that persistent Epstein-Barr virus infection is a possibility.

"The Postviral Fatigue Syndrome—An Analysis of the Findings in 50 Cases." by P. O. Behan et al. *Journal of Infection*, Vol. 10, 1988. In this Scottish medical journal, authors review fifty cases of postviral fatigue, with a particular look at immunological and virological tests. Findings confirm the existence of an organic disorder.

"Coping With Chronic Fatigue Syndrome." By Helen Grierson et al. *Patient Care*, November 15, 1987. Overview on CFS, with a particular focus on how primary-care physicians can manage the disorder in their practices.

"Phenotypic and Functional Deficiency of Natural Killer Cells in Patients with Chronic Fatigue Syndrome." By Michael Caligiuri et al. *The Journal of Immunology*, November 15, 1987. This highly technical article pinpoints a measurable immunological disorder in CFS patients. Researchers find they often have below-normal levels of natural killer cells, which are important in combatting viral infections.

"Chronic Fatigue Syndrome and the Diagnostic Utility of Antibody to Epstein-Barr Virus Early Antigen." By Dr. Walter C. Hellinger et al. *Journal of American Medicine*, August 19, 1988. Authors dispute theory that certain Epstein-Barr virus antibodies are a sign of chronic fatigue syndrome and conclude the antibody test has no diagnostic value.

"T-Cell Lymphomas Containing Epstein-Barr Viral DNA in Patients with Chronic Epstein-Barr Virus Infections." By Dr. James F. Jones et al. *New England Journal of Medicine*, March 24, 1988. Authors report on three fatal cancer cases in patients with chronic Epstein-Barr virus infections. The study broadens previous understanding of how the virus works but does not clearly suggest a heightened risk of cancer among CFS patients.

"A Cluster of Patients With Chronic Mononucleosis-Like Syndrome: Is Epstein-Barr Virus the Cause?" By Dr. Gary Holmes et al. *Journal of American Medicine*, May 1, 1987. At the request of physicians Paul Cheney and Daniel Peterson, Centers for Disease Control scientists came to Incline Village, Nevada, to study the reported epidemic. They conclude here that the Epstein-Barr virus can not clearly be implicated.

"Frequency of 'Chronic Active Epstein-Barr Virus Infection' In a General Medical Practice." By Dr. Dedra Buchwald et al. *Journal of American Medicine,* May 1, 1987.
Study found that 21 percent of 500 randomly selected patients seeking care in a general medical practice were suffering from a syndrome resembling that described as chronic active Epstein-Barr virus infection.

"Chronic Epstein-Barr Virus Infection." By Dr. James F. Jones and Dr. Stephen E. Straus. *Annual Review of Medicine,* Vol. 38, 1987.
A look at the biology of the Epstein-Barr virus, the normal host immunological response, and the clinical manifestations of infection. Treatment options and the process through which the virus is reactivated are also covered.

"Acyclovir Treatment of a Chronic Fatigue Syndrome With Unusual EBV Serologic Profiles: Lack of Efficacy in a Controlled Trial." By Dr. Stephen E. Straus et al. *Clinical Research,* Vol. 35, 1987.
Report on a double-blind study using acyclovir with chronic fatigue syndrome that concludes the drug is no more effective than using a placebo.

"Allergy and the Syndrome of Chronic Epstein-Barr Virus Infection." By Dr. Robert C. Welliver. *Journal of Allergy and Clinical Immunology,* August 1986.
Author reviews evidence that allergies are associated with CEBV infection and may be one cause. Two other more technical articles report on specific studies in the same journal.

"Gamma Globulin Therapy of Chronic Mononucleosis Syndrome." By Dr. Richard Eugene DuBois. *AIDS Research,* Vol. 2, Supplement 1, 1986.
This review of the use of gamma globulin in the treatment of the disorder concludes that it is often effective.

"Characteristic T Cell Dysfunction in Patients with Chronic Active Epstein-Barr Virus Infection." By Giovanna Tosato et al. *The Journal of Immunology,* May 1985.
Suppressed T cell activity (which suggests diminished capacity to combat infection) was observed in patients with chronic Epstein-Barr virus infection.

"Evidence for Active Epstein-Barr Virus Infection in Patients with Persistent, Unexplained Illnesses: Elevated Anti-Early Antigen

Antibodies." By Dr. James F. Jones et al. *Annals of Internal Medicine*, January 1985.
"Persisting Illness and Fatigue in Adults with Evidence of Epstein-Barr Virus Infection." By Dr. Stephen E. Straus et al.
"Chronicity of Epstein-Barr Virus Infection," an editorial by Dr. James C. Niederman. *Annals of Internal Medicine*, January, 1985.
"Chronic Mononucleosis Syndrome." By Dr. Richard DuBois. *Southern Medical Journal*, November 1984.
All four articles explore the possibility that the Epstein-Barr virus causes the lingering illness we now know as chronic fatigue syndrome. They were among the earliest to call scientific attention to the problem.

Books

Many excellent books provide useful information to CFS patients. Some focus specifically on the syndrome; others discuss related symptoms, such as balance disorders, phobias, and yeast infections. Descriptions of diagnostic tests, medications, and alternative therapies also serve as key reference sources for people with CFS. A sampling of the best, including many that provided valuable information for this book, are listed below.

CFIDS: The Disease of a Thousand Names. By Dr. David S. Bell. Pollard Publications. 1991.
Discussion of chronic fatigue syndrome, including a technical explanation of the mechanisms that may cause it. Several chapters are written to help physicians treat their patients.

What Really Killed Gilda Radner? Frontline Reports on the CFS Epidemic. By Neenyah Ostrom. That New Magazine Inc. 1991.
Long-time writer for the *New York Native* provides a look at the politics of the chronic fatigue syndrome movement.

CFIDS: An Owner's Manual by Barbara Brooks and Nancy Smith. 1988. (Available from Barbara Brooks & Nancy Smith, Box 6456, Silver Spring, Maryland 20906.)
Self-published handbook written by two CFS patients. The primary focus is on the debilitating social and emotional consequences of the illness and how to cope with them.

"Chronic Fatigue Syndrome: A Personal Diary." By Arnold H. Goldberg, M.D. (Available from Dr. A. H. Goldberg, 920 King St.
West, Kitchener, Ontario, Canada N2G 1G4.)
Spiral-bound workbook that enables patients to keep records of their
medical history, to list visits to physicians, and to monitor treatments
and medications received. Sections are available to describe relapses,
chart the ups and downs of the illness on a daily basis, and assess
monthly progress.

The Mile-High Staircase. By Toni Jeffreys. Hodder and Stoughton,
1982. (Available from ANZME, P.O. Box 35–429, Browns Bay
Auckland 10, New Zealand)
The moving story of an Australian women's struggle with chronic
fatigue syndrome, known overseas as myalgic encephalomyelitis.

*Chronic Fatigue Syndrome: A Victim's Guide to Understanding, Treating,
and Coping With This Debilitating Illness* by Gregg Charles Fisher.
Warner Books, 1989.
Personal story of a young divinity student and his wife who have been
unusually sick with CFS for almost ten years. Includes essays from
medical experts.

Chronic Fatigue Syndrome: The Hidden Epidemic by Jesse Stoff, M.D. and
Charles Pellegrino. Random House, 1988.
One doctor's treatment regimen, which is rooted in a strong belief in
the mind–body connection and the conviction that liver-related problems are the source of much of the dysfunction.

"Social Security Benefits and Chronic Fatigue Syndrome." By Samuel
J. Imperati and Janis Pearson. (Available from: CFIDS Society,
Box 230108, Portland, Oregon 97223.)
A booklet written specifically for CFS patients that covers the applications
and hearings process for obtaining Social Security disability benefits.

Social Security Disability Benefits: How to Get Them! How to Keep Them!
By James W. Ross. (Available from Ross Publishing Co., 188
Forrester Rd., Slippery Rock, Pennsylvania 16057, or the CFIDS
Society, Box 230108, Portland, Oregon 97223.)
Another excellent resource on applying for Social Security disability.

Physicians' Desk Reference. Publisher, Edward R. Barnhart. Medical
Economics Co. Annual publication.
A standard reference book for physicians, *PDR* describes 2,000 major
pharmaceutical and diagnostic products, along with recommended use,

appropriate dosage, possible adverse reactions, and appropriate precautions. Although *PDR* is somewhat technical, it is an invaluable resource.

The People's Book of Medical Tests. By David S. Sobel, M.D. and Tom Ferguson, M.D. Summit Books, 1985.

The Patient's Guide to Medical Tests. By Cathey Pinckney and Edward R. Pinckney, M.D. Facts on File, 1986.
Geared to the health care consumer, both books describe hundreds of common diagnostic medical tests, including many that can be done at home. Readily accessible to the layperson, they describe how and why each test is performed, how it feels, what risks are associated with it, and what the results mean.

The New People's Pharmacy. By Joe Graedon. Bantam and Graedon Enterprises, 1985.
Opinionated guide to effective medications—and why ineffective ones are sometimes pushed instead. Author covers prescription and over-the-counter drugs, particularly emphasizing pain relief, antiviral medication, drugs for the heart and blood pressure, and what's coming in the years ahead.

The Essential Guide to Prescription Drugs 1988. By James W. Long. Harper & Row, 1988.

The Essential Guide to Nonprescription Drugs. By David R. Zimmerman. Harper & Row, 1983.
Consumer-oriented information about commonly used prescription and over-the-counter drugs.

Free Yourself from Pain. By Dr. David E. Bresler with Richard Trubo. A Fireside Book by Simon & Schuster, 1979.
Techniques for defeating chronic pain. Authors cover causes of pain, traditional remedies, including drugs and surgery, exercise therapies, and unconventional techniques. The power of inner healing is also explored.

The Natural Family Doctor: The Comprehensive Self-Help Guide to Health and Natural Medicine. By Dr. Andrew Stanway with Richard Grossman. A Fireside Book by Simon & Schuster, 1987.
Thorough, informative discussions on a range of healing techniques beyond the purview of orthodox medicine. Health maintenance—including diet, exercise, breathing techniques, and relaxation—are

discussed. Among the specific therapies described are homeopathy, herbalism, hydrotherapy, chiropractic, massage, reflexology, yoga, therapeutic touch, hypnotherapy, meditation, and biofeedback.

Seeing with the Mind's Eye: The History, Techniques and Uses of Visualization. By Dr. Mike Samuels and Nancy Samuels. Random House and Bookworks, 1977.
A fascinating look at the uses of visualization as a tool for healing and as a mode of releasing creativity.

Well Body Book. By Mike Samuels and Hall Bennet. Random House and Bookworks, 1973.
A classic in the realm of holistic healing techniques. A patient workbook that focuses on well-being and the prevention of disease, with an emphasis on the capacity to assume a greater control over your own health. Although it includes some information about specific diseases, its focus is on prevention.

Jane Brody's Nutrition Book. By Jane Brody. Bantam Books, 1987.
Commonsense guide to the principles of sound nutrition. Although the author's guidelines are not geared specifically to ailing people, her recommendations are sensible and widely relevant.

The Yeast Connection. By William Crook, M.D. Professional Books, 1983.
Bestselling book that popularized the theory that yeast infections—brought on by poor diet, excessive use of antibiotics, and other environmental toxins—cause a wide range of illnesses.

Coping with Your Allergies. By Natalie Golos and Frances Golos Globitz. A Fireside book by Simon & Schuster, 1986.
A guide to clinical ecology, how allergies cause illness, and what to do about them.

The New Allergy Guide Book. By Dr. Harry Swartz. Continuum, 1987.
A practical program of prevention and control. Explains the cause of allergies, discusses the link between the emotions and allergy, and emphasizes ways to prevent or minimize the onset of allergic reactions.

Balancing Act: A Handbook for People with Dizziness and Balance Disorders. By Mary Ann Watson and Helen Sinclair.
Illustrated guide written for the lay patient, it examines balance disorders, which often afflict chronic fatigue syndrome patients, in simple language and discusses available treatment. Dietary suggestions are included.

Phobia Free. By Dr. Harold N. Levinson with Steven Carter. M. Evans and Co., 1986.
An invaluable guide for chronic fatigue syndrome patients who suffer from panic attacks. Levinson argues that most irrational phobias have a physiological basis—usually linked to inner-ear dysfunction—and can be treated easily.

The Consumer Health Information Source Book. By Alan M. Rees and Jodith Janes. R. R. Bowker Co., 1984.
Comprehensive guide to sources of health care information. Includes general-interest and specialized bibliographies, lists of health magazines, newsletters and consumer publications, and books and pamphlets on scores of topics, including medical consumerism, physical fitness and self-health care, women's health, mental health, headaches, allergies, and neurological diseases.

The Self-Help Sourcebook: Finding and Forming Mutual Aid Self-Help Groups. (Available from Self-Help Clearinghouse, St. Clares-Riverside Medical Center, Pocono Road, Denville, New Jersey 07834.)
A directory of more than 500 model self-help groups covering a broad range of addictions, disabilities, and illness. Includes general how-to's for starting self-help groups, contacts for self-help clearinghouses worldwide, and a listing of toll-free national help lines.

Appendix D:
Glossary

Allergen. Any substance that provokes a hypersensitive, or allergic, reaction in the body; pollen, house dust, plants, and animal dander are common allergens.

Allergy. A disorder in which a susceptible individual launches an immunological response against a normally harmless foreign substance; an allergic response can include swelling, sneezing, rash, breathing difficulties, and many other symptoms.

Antibody. Specialized protein molecule produced by the lymph tissue as part of a normal immunological response to destroy or neutralize a specific toxin or foreign substance (antigen) that has invaded the body.

Antidepressant. One of a class of pharmaceutical products used to alleviate or prevent the symptoms of depression.

Antigen. A foreign substance that the body combats by producing an antibody.

Antihistamine. Class of drugs used to reduce the effects of histamines, which are released by the body during an allergic reaction.

Arthralgia. Joint pain, especially unaccompanied by inflammation.

Assay. Test or trial; a drug assay is used to determine potency, purity, efficacy or appropriate dosage of a medication.

Autoimmune disease. Condition in which the immune system mistakes body cells and tissues for enemy invaders and launches an attack against them. The cause of most autoimmune diseases, including multiple sclerosis, lupus, thyroiditis, and rheumatoid arthritis, is not known. Some researchers believe CFS is an autoimmune disease.

Candidiasis. Yeast-like infection caused by the *Candida albicans* fungus that generally appears in moist areas of the body, including the mouth and vagina, as well as in the folds of the skin and under the nails. In rare circumstances, the infection can spread throughout the body.

Cell transformation. Process by which a virus infects a human cell and tinkers with its DNA, so that every time the cell replicates, the virus is also reproduced.

Chronic fatigue immune dysfunction syndrome (CFIDS). Another name for chronic fatigue syndrome, it is preferred by some patient groups and physicians because it suggests an immunological component to the disorder.

Clinical immunology. Study of the human immune system as applied in a medical practice.

Cofactors. Factors that do not cause disease alone but that can intensify the effects of other causative factors; stress, for example, can be a cofactor in viral disease.

Cognitive dysfunction. Abnormal problems with the absorption, retention, or use of knowledge, judgment, or the ability to learn and think.

Contagion. Transmission of disease from an afflicted person to a healthy one.

Cytokines. Naturally occurring hormones produced by human cells in the course of an immunological response to infection. Lymphokines and interleukins are particular types of cytokines.

Endocrinology. Branch of medical science that studies the body's endocrine, or hormonal, system.

Endogenous depression. Type of depression that originates from within the body, as when there is a chemical imbalance; it contrasts with exogenous depression, which is not physiological in origin.

Epidemic. Sudden and rapidly spreading outbreak of disease affecting a significant number of people in one location at the same time.

Epidemiology. Branch of medical science that studies the pattern of disease in a population, including its spread, incidence, and means of control.

Epstein-Barr virus. One of the herpes family of viruses, EBV causes chronic mononucleosis and several rare forms of cancer. The activated virus is no longer thought to cause chronic fatigue syndrome but is often a sign of it.

Exogenous depression. Reactive depression; a type of depression that has its origins outside the body and is often caused by emotional factors.

Gastrointestinal. Of or relating to the stomach and the intestines.

Hematologic. Relating to blood or blood-forming tissues.

Hepatic. Relating to the liver.

Herpes viruses. Family of viruses that can remain latent in the body for years; once infected, human beings carry herpes viruses for life; the six known herpes viruses are herpes simplex I, herpes simplex II, Epstein-Barr, cytomegalovirus, varicella zoster, and human herpesvirus-6.

Human Herpesvirus-6. One of the herpes family of viruses, HHV6 was discovered in 1986; the virus infects immune system cells but it is not yet known to cause a specific disease.

Immune complex. Molecule formed by the binding of an antigen and an antibody that can cause inflammation and is often involved in autoimmune disease.

Immune system. System of defense by which the body protects itself against bacteria, virus, pollutants, and other foreign invaders.

Immunoglobulin (Ig). One of the five classes of antibodies that respond to foreign invaders. IgM antibodies generally appear early in an immune response while IgG antibodies appear later. IgA antibodies are concentrated in the gastrointestinal and respiratory tracts as well as in secretions. IgE antibodies are involved in allergic response. IgD antibodies are still poorly understood.

Infectious mononucleosis. "Kissing disease of adolescence," acute mono is caused by the Epstein-Barr virus and is transmitted via saliva; CFS and mono share many of the same symptoms.

Interferon. Lymphokine that plays a key role in immune system response by stimulating the production of macrophages, B cells, and certain T cells and helping to regulate the manufacture of antibodies.

Interleukin. Protein that plays a crucial role in proper immune system response. In the course of fighting an infection, this protein can actually produce fever and other flu-like symptoms.

Latent. Used in virology to describe a dormant period when a virus is detectable but inactive.

Lymphocyte. Subgroup of white blood cells that originate in the body's lymphoid tissues and glands and play an important role in immune system response. B lymphocyte cells produce the antibodies to combat antigens whereas T lymphocyte cells can destroy antigens directly.

Lymphokines. Hormones produced by the T lymphocytes to stimulate immune system response, particularly the production of macrophages, B lymphocytes, and other T cells.

Lymphoma. Tumor of the lymph tissues that is usually malignant.

Lysing virus. Type of virus that damages or destroys the membrane of its host cell in order to escape into the bloodstream.

Macrophages. Frontline immune system cells programmed to surround and ingest dead tissues and cellular debris. A subclass of phagocytes found in the liver, spleen, and loose connective tissue.

Multiple sclerosis. Autoimmune disease characterized by the damage to the nerve fibers of the brain and spinal cord. MS progresses over time, sometimes causing paralysis, tremors, and numbness.

Myalgia. Muscular pain.

Myalgic encephalomyelitis. Another name for chronic fatigue syndrome, in widespread use in Great Britain and elsewhere in Europe.

Natural killer cells. Cells of the immune system programmed to disintegrate tumor or virus-infected cells. Below-normal levels of NK cells have been pinpointed in many CFS patients.

Neurology. Branch of medical science that deals with the human nervous system, including the brain and the spinal cord.

Neuromyasthenia. Disease of the nerves and muscles; the word is sometimes used as a synonym for chronic fatigue syndrome.

Neurotransmitters. Chemical substances released from the nerve endings to transmit messages across synapses to other nerves.

Phagocytes. Scavenger cells of the human immune system that ingest bacteria, protozoa, cellular debris, and other foreign particles.

Photophobia. Undue sensitivity to light.

Placebo. Inert substance without pharmaceutical benefits that may still be useful for treating illness because of a patient's belief in its efficacy. When new drugs are tested, placebos are often administered to control groups as a means of comparison.

Premorbid. Prior to illness.

Psychoneuroimmunology. Branch of science that studies the links between the human nervous and immunological systems and seeks a biochemical basis for the mind–body connection.

Prognosis. Likely course of a disease and the prospect for recovery, as determined by the experience of previous cases and the condition of the patient.

Reactivation. Process by which a latent virus emerges from dormancy to cause new infection or illness.

Relapse. Worsening of the signs and symptoms of illness after a period of apparent improvement.

Retrovirus. A class of viruses with the unusual property of transmitting information in a backward flow from RNA to DNA. Recent research says a retrovirus may be associated with CFS.

Scotomata. Area within the field of vision in which sight is absent or impaired.

Self-limiting. Disease that by its very nature runs its course and then resolves, often without treatment.

Sign. Objective indicator of a physical disorder as measured by a doctor; contrast with symptom, which refers to a patient's complaint.

Symptom. Subjective indicator of a physical disorder as cited by a patient; an indication of illness that cannot be measured.

Syndrome. Constellation of signs and symptoms that is clinically distinct but that may represent a group of diseases and be caused by more than one factor.

Systemic lupus erythematosus. Autoimmune disease commonly known as lupus that causes inflammation of the skin and internal organs, adversely affecting the blood vessels and kidneys and sometimes causing tumors of the skin and nervous system.

Thyroiditis. Inflammation of the thyroid gland; the chronic condition is an autoimmune disorder.

Titer. Concentration of antibodies produced against a particular antigen.

Vestibular system. System of balance controlled by the inner ear.

Index